Contents

KV-702-461

List of Tables

List of Figures

Page 4

Glossary of Terms

Accreditation: Accreditation may be either professional or academic. Professional accreditation is the process by which a professional body certifies and recognises an educational course as meeting the requirements of professional registration. Academic accreditation refers to the process by which an academic body accredits a course of study leading to a recognised award such as a degree. In some institutions this process is also referred to as validation.

An Bord Altranais: Statutory regulatory body for nursing and midwifery established under the Nurses Act 1985.

Clinical Learning Environment: The environment in which clinical learning takes place.

Clinical Placement: An approved learning experience that provides nursing students with the practice elements of the nursing degree programme.

Clinical Placement Co-ordinator: Practice-based nurse who co-ordinates nursing students' clinical learning placements.

Clinical Nurse Manager: Clinical nurse engaged in the management of clinical nursing services.

Degree Programme: Four-year pre-registration degree programme leading to registration as a nurse.

Divisions of Register: Categories of nursing personnel registerable with An Bord Altranais, namely general, psychiatric, mental handicap, midwifery, sick children's, public health nursing and nurse tutors.

EU Directives: European Directives that regulate the minimum number of hours required related to theoretical and clinical learning in programmes leading to registration as a nurse within the European Union.

Mature Applicant: A person who attained the age of 23 years on the first day of January of the year in which s/he was admitted to a course leading to an award.

Nurse Practice Development Co-ordinator: Practice-based nurse with responsibility for leading and directing developments in nursing practice within a health service provider.

Nurse Tutor: Nurses who have undertaken a specific course leading to registration as a nurse tutor and whose names are on the register of nurse tutors maintained by An Bord Altranais.

Preceptor: A registered nurse who has been specially prepared to guide and direct student learning during clinical placement. A preceptor is an experienced nurse, midwife or community nurse within a practice placement who acts as a role model and resource for a student who is assigned to him or her for a specific time span or experience.

Register: The register of nurses maintained by An Bord Altranais pursuant to the Nurses Act 1985.

Rostered Placement: The element of the nursing degree programme during which the nursing student is employed by the service provider.

Service Provider: Providers of health, welfare, social and educational services who will provide the clinical learning component of the four-year pre-registration degree programme.

Service User: Any user of the services described above including patients / clients and their significant others.

Glossary of Terms

Stakeholders: Those parties including An Bord Altranais, the Department of Health and Children, the Department of Education and Science, the Department of Finance, Higher Education Authority (HEA), National Council for Educational Awards, third-level institutions, health service providers and students involved in the four-year pre-registration degree programme. Patients / service users are also included as stakeholders when appropriate. The National Qualifications Authority, when established, will be included amongst the stakeholders.

Standard Applicant: An applicant to nursing who applies for entry through the normal application process on the basis of his or her school leaving qualifications.

Supernumerary: Nursing student not included in the rostered complement of nurses who are employed by health service providers.

Third-level Institutions: Institutions providing third-level education including Universities, Institutes of Technology and Colleges of Education.

Executive Summary
and Summary of Recommendations

Executive Summary

In its report *A Blueprint for the Future* (1998), the Commission on Nursing recommended the establishment of the Nursing Education Forum to the Minister for Health and Children.

The Forum, which was established in February 1999, included the stakeholders in health service provision and education in Ireland (it comprised thirty-four nominated representatives from various organisations active in nursing education in Ireland and an independent chair). Its primary objective was to develop a strategic framework for the introduction of a pre-registration nursing degree programme in general, psychiatric and mental handicap nursing.

Four working principles guided the Forum in the development of this strategy. They were: partnership; consultation; openness and transparency; and adherence to the spirit and letter of the report of the Commission on Nursing in relation to pre-registration nursing education in Ireland.

This strategy for nursing education is based on the World Health Organisation's *Nurses and Midwives for Health, A WHO European Strategy for Nursing and Midwifery Education* (1999). It is also informed by the publications of An Bord Altranais and its view on the role and function of the nurse. The strategy developed by the Forum contains over forty recommendations on the implementation of the four-year pre-registration nursing degree programme, which the Forum believes are achievable in the short to medium term.

The Forum points out that the transition to a pre-registration nursing degree programme will involve considerable change which will require a proactive and sustained approach from the stakeholders. The common thread throughout this strategy is "partnership". A close and committed partnership between all stakeholders at all stages of the transition is required if the implementation programme is to be a success. In the formulation of this strategy, Forum members worked together in partnership to develop a common vision for the future pre-registration nursing degree programme. Local stakeholders involved in the delivery of each pre-registration nursing degree programme should also work together to develop a common shared vision.

The Forum believes that students graduating from the pre-registration nursing degree programme should be professional nurses who are safe, caring, competent decision makers, willing to accept personal and professional accountability for evidence-based practice. It considers that nurse graduates should be flexible, adaptable and reflective practitioners, integral members of the multi-disciplinary team and should adopt a life-long approach to learning.

The Forum recognises that the successful recruitment and selection of nursing students is vital to the delivery of healthcare and that this can only be carried out effectively by health service providers and third-level academic institutions working closely in partnership.

After studying in detail all procedures for selecting nursing students, the Forum concludes that the selection process utilised should be based on the principles of transparency, impartiality and efficiency and must be capable of securing the support of both the profession and the general public. It recommends that the assessment test and the interview for school leavers be discontinued from 2001 when the nursing application system is transferred to the Central Applications Office (CAO).

This change, as with the other changes in application procedures and selection systems over the past decade, could lead to some confusion amongst potential applicants, their parents and teachers. To ensure clarity about the process of selecting nursing students, the Forum recommends a co-ordinated promotional and marketing campaign to maintain the number of applicants. While recommending that An Bord Altranais continues to co-ordinate and provide strategic direction to the promotion and marketing of nursing as a career, it recognises that overall promotion and marketing of nursing is a shared responsibility between the stakeholders.

Given that the proportion of mature applicants for nursing education programmes rose from 14% in 1997 to 29% in 2000, and that current demographic trends indicate that the number of school leavers is expected to drop in the future, the Forum points out that consideration must be given to attracting mature applicants to the profession. While the Commission on Nursing recommended that a quota of places for mature students be established in each third-level institution providing pre-registration nursing education programmes, the Forum recommends that discussions on the framework for the bursary / sponsorship system for mature nursing student applicants should commence as soon as possible between the Department of Health and Children, An Bord Altranais and the health service providers. It also recommends that the third-level institutions and health service providers take steps to prepare and support mature students selected to undertake the pre-registration nursing degree programme.

The Forum notes that the transition to the pre-registration degree programme must be actively managed at all stages of the process to ensure that all stakeholders are fully informed and committed to the change. A clear understanding of the areas of authority and competence, and the consequent roles and responsibilities of each stakeholder needs to be established at both national and local levels. The Forum therefore recommends that before 2002, a memorandum of understanding be drawn up and signed by stakeholders at local level between each third-level institution and its related health service providers.

To facilitate the change to a degree-based programme, the Forum points out that those involved in the transition process must consider and understand the existing structures within Irish healthcare, third-level institutions and related organisations. The most effective means of managing change is by establishing structures that give concrete expression to partnership and ensure a formal and networked monitoring, evaluation and feedback system. To facilitate this process, the Forum recommends that formal structures should be put in place.

A national implementation committee is recommended to oversee the implementation of the degree programme. The committee membership should represent all the relevant stakeholders in nursing education. It should have an independent chair, nominated by the Minister for Health and Children, in consultation with the Minister for Education and Science. The Forum recommends that the national implementation committee should be established as soon as possible, its initial task being to prepare a plan of the processes and actions necessary to ensure the implementation of the Forum's recommendations in a structured, co-ordinated and coherent manner.

An inter-departmental steering committee is also recommended, its primary function being to co-ordinate the activities and policies of the Departments of Health and Children and Education and Science during the transition to a degree programme. The inter-departmental committee should comprise representatives of the Departments of Health and Children, Education and Science, and Finance and the Higher Education Authority.

The Forum also recommends that local joint working groups on nursing education be established comprising representatives of a third-level educational institution providing pre-registration nursing education and its associated health service providers. Their purpose would be to provide a strategic overview of the change process, monitor progress and address such partnership issues as may arise. To ensure that formal structures for partnership at a local level are maintained, it is recommended that the groups should remain in existence after the transition is complete.

The Forum attaches great importance to communicating developments as they happen. At each level of implementation, the Forum holds that there is a responsibility to communicate on developments in nursing education to relevant stakeholders. The Forum recommends that the national implementation committee, inter-departmental steering committee and local joint working groups should each draw up and implement a strategy for communication with their relevant stakeholders. The objective should be to ensure that those who will be affected by the proposed changes are fully briefed on the reasons and rationale for the change and have the opportunity to discuss their possible implications.

Curriculum design for pre-registration nursing education must take place within the regulatory framework of An Bord Altranais' requirements and standards and EU Directives. The Forum notes that the reactions to the introduction of the diploma programme informed its decision to advocate an approach to curriculum design based on the principles of flexibility; eclecticism; transferability and progression; utility; evidence base and shared learning.

The Forum points out that the NEATE report identified that the curriculum for the diploma programme was being centrally imposed and as a result there was insufficient flexibility in it to allow adaptation to local needs. The Forum considers that its principles-based approach acts as a guide to curriculum design, which can be interpreted locally.

In order to ensure a quality education for nursing students, the Forum feels strongly that all relevant stakeholders should be actively involved in the development, design and evaluation of the curriculum.

Learning the practice of nursing is an integral part of the nursing curriculum and the establishment of structures to support student learning in the clinical learning environment, the Forum points out, is essential.

It is felt strongly that nursing students need exposure to practice through a range of placements in different settings where care is delivered. The task of organising this is significant and requires considerable planning and co-ordination between third-level institutions and health service providers. The Forum therefore recommends that an allocation function be established in each third-level institution to co-ordinate clinical learning placements and that an individual from each health service provider liaise with the responsible person in the third-level institution in relation to clinical placement allocations.

It is crucial to the success and integrity of the nursing degree programme that clinical staff are adequately prepared for their teaching roles. The Forum recommends that stakeholders should ensure that within five years of the commencement of the degree programme all nurses who support students have attended a teaching and assessing course if they have not already done so.

The clinical placement will provide the nursing student with support and learning opportunities to facilitate the practice of nursing. There are a range of key individuals with whom nursing students will interact directly.

The preceptor is a registered nurse who develops a relationship with, acts as a role model to, and works closely with the student throughout the placement. The Forum recommends that each student on placement should be assigned a named preceptor who is a registered nurse. The clinical nurse manager has an important role in creating and maintaining a clinical learning environment. The Forum recommends that this role continue to be recognised and supported. Clinical placement co-ordinators were introduced as a mechanism to support students on placement during the introduction of the diploma programme. The Commission on Nursing recommended that the role be evaluated and this study was in progress as the Forum concluded its deliberations. The Forum recommends that the role be retained, but that it may be redefined once the results of the study are known. Teaching

staff from third-level institutions are also key in facilitating and contributing to the clinical learning of students.

As also recommended in the report of the Commission on Nursing, the Forum recommends the development of joint appointments and other innovative strategies to develop partnership between third-level institutions and health service providers. The precise nature and role of such appointments should be agreed within local partnerships.

The Forum estimates that the average cost per annum of the degree programme will be £5,300 per student and the total revenue cost will be £57 million in 2002 prices. The additional revenue cost of the degree programme, once the diploma costs are offset against it, is estimated at £12.2 million, an increase of 25% compared to the diploma programme. A preliminary estimate of the capital investment required is £135 million.

Over the past nineteen months, the Nursing Education Forum has recognised at first hand the range of opportunities and challenges that face nursing. Partnership between all stakeholders is a key requisite as nursing develops and meets the ever changing needs of society. Through the work of the Forum partnership has been enhanced at a strategic level. It is critical that this continues, to ensure that nursing can flourish and respond appropriately to the range of issues facing the Irish health sector.

Summary of Recommendations

Chapter 2

- The Forum recommends that local stakeholders involved in the delivery of each pre-registration nursing degree programme should work in partnership to develop a common shared vision for nursing education.

Chapter 3

- The Forum recommends that the assessment test and the interview for school leavers be discontinued from 2001 under the transfer of the application system to the CAO.
- The Forum recommends that An Bord Altranais monitor and review on a continuing basis the issue of the separate CAO lists for nursing.
- The Forum recommends that An Bord Altranais continue to co-ordinate and provide strategic direction to the promotion and marketing of nursing as a career.
- The Forum recommends that An Bord Altranais undertake further research to examine the rationale for, and impact of, maintaining three points of access to pre-registration nursing.
- The Forum recommends that An Bord Altranais monitor the impact of the withdrawal of the non-means tested grant.
- The Forum recommends that discussions on the framework for a bursary/ sponsorship system for mature nursing students commence as soon as possible between the Department of Health and Children, An Bord Altranais and health service providers.

- The Forum recommends that third-level institutions and health service providers make provision for the support that mature students will require to undertake the pre-registration nursing degree programme.

Chapter 4

- The Forum recommends that, before 2002, a memorandum of understanding be drawn up and signed by stakeholders at local level between each third-level institution and its related health service providers.
- The Forum recommends that appropriate academic structures for a nursing degree programme be established within each third-level institution such as a faculty, school or department of nursing. A nurse at an appropriate grade consistent with other academic departments should head this faculty, school or department of nursing.
- The Forum recommends the establishment of a national implementation committee to oversee the implementation of the pre-registration nursing degree programme.
- The Forum recommends that the national implementation committee should be established as soon as possible and funded by the Department of Health and Children. Its initial task should be to prepare a plan of the processes and actions necessary to ensure the implementation of the Forum's recommendations in a structured, co-ordinated and coherent manner in compliance with the timescale set out in this report. The Forum recommends that the Minister for Health and Children,

following consultation with the Minister for Education and Science, appoint an independent chair and the members of the national implementation committee.

- The Forum recommends that an inter-departmental steering committee should be established to co-ordinate the activities and policies of the Departments of Health and Children and Education and Science during the transition to a degree programme.

- The Forum recommends that the inter-departmental steering committee should comprise representatives of the Departments of Health and Children, Education and Science, Finance and the Higher Education Authority.

- The Forum recommends that local joint working groups on nursing education be established comprising representatives of a third-level educational institution providing pre-registration nursing education and its associated health service providers.

- The Forum recommends that the local joint working groups on nursing education should remain in existence after the transition is complete.

- The Forum recommends that formal induction programmes be provided by the third-level institutions to facilitate the transfer and integration of nurse teachers into the third-level sector.

- The Forum recommends that one individual should be designated as project manager of the transition to the degree programme for the duration of the transition process by each local joint working group on nursing education.

- The Forum recommends that the national implementation committee,

inter-departmental steering committee and local joint working groups should each draw up and implement a strategy for communication with their relevant stakeholders and each other.

- The Forum recommends that the inter-departmental steering committee undertake, as a matter of priority, a detailed analysis for each third-level institution, of the necessary capital investment required. In addition, the Forum recommends that every reasonable effort be made to facilitate the full physical integration of nursing students within third-level institutions at the earliest practicable date.

- The Forum recommends that all nursing students, both diploma and degree, and those nurse teachers who wish to move into third-level should be fully integrated into the third-level system in time for the start of the degree programme in 2002.

Chapter 5

- The Forum recommends that discussion on the model of professional education to underpin the nursing degree programme should take place between third-level institutions and health service providers.

- The Forum recommends that the curriculum design be dynamic and flexible to permit responsiveness to local needs.

- The Forum recommends that the curriculum design for the nursing degree programme be eclectic insofar as it draws on knowledge from diverse sources and uses a variety of teaching/learning strategies.

- The Forum recommends that research be undertaken by An Bord Altranais to examine the issues pertaining to transferability and progression of nursing education programmes leading to registration.

- The Forum recommends that a flexible and dynamic approach be adopted to facilitate the transfer and progression of students as far as practicable and suggests that this be considered on an individual basis.

- The Forum recommends that in the development of curricula for the new four-year degree programme in pre-registration nursing education in Ireland, the National Qualifications Authority and all third-level institutions providing nursing education programmes should ensure that there are transfer pathways in place, thereby enabling nursing students to have the option of changing course specialty, or even to transfer to programmes outside of nursing.

- The Forum recommends that clinical placements should be undertaken early in the programme and there should be reflective time built into the rostered year to enhance the consolidation of theory and practice.

- The Forum recommends that the curriculum design for the pre-registration nursing degree programme should have a sound theoretical base.

- The Forum recommends that nursing students should be actively encouraged to learn with and from other healthcare professionals.

- The Forum recommends that to ensure a quality education for nursing students all stakeholders, including the students themselves, should be actively involved in the evaluation of the pre-registration nursing degree programme.

Chapter 6

- The Forum recommends that an allocations function be established in each third-level institution to co-ordinate the placement of students for clinical learning.

- The Forum recommends that a designated person within each health service provider should be given responsibility to liaise with the responsible person within the third-level institution in relation to clinical placement allocations.

- The Forum recommends that decisions on the allocation of rostered placements should involve particularly close consultation between third-level institutions and health service providers.

- The Forum recommends a pilot project to explore the need for the clinical placement co-ordinator post within community healthcare.

- The Forum recommends that health service providers, in partnership with the relevant third-level institution, should ensure that nurses who support students have attended a teaching and assessing course. It further recommends that within five years of the start of the degree programme all nurses who support students and who have not already completed such a course should have done so.

- The Forum recommends that each student whilst on clinical placement should be assigned a named preceptor who is a registered nurse.

- The Forum recommends that the clinical nurse manager continue to have a pivotal role in creating and maintaining a clinical learning environment.

- The Forum recommends that the role of clinical placement co-ordinator be retained and that the role may be redefined depending on the final results of role evaluation.

- The Forum recommends that third-level institutions examine opportunities and develop innovative strategies for nurse lecturers to develop their links with clinical areas.
- The Forum recommends the development of joint appointments and other innovative strategies to enhance partnership between third-level institutions and health service providers, the precise role and nature of which should be agreed within local partnerships.
- The Forum recommends that within the clinical learning environment all involved should devise innovative and effective ways to maximise the opportunity for students to reflect on and learn from their clinical experience. The Forum recommends that specific periods of protected time be identified for reflection during supernumerary and rostered placements. The amount of time allocated should be agreed formally between third-level institutions and health service providers and included in the memorandum of understanding.

Chapter 7

- The Forum recommends that the Department of Health and Children engage external consultants at the earliest opportunity to examine in detail the student-staff ratio during the twelve-month rostered clinical placement.
- The Forum recommends that priority be accorded by health service providers to the provision of preceptorship training for clinical nursing staff. If the existing resources are inadequate for this purpose, then a case should be made by individual providers to the Department of Health and Children for additional funding for this particular form of training, based on an analysis of existing expenditure on continuing nursing education.
- The Forum recommends that discussions should take place between the Departments of Finance and Health and Children and health service providers on the extent, if any, to which funding on student meals may be offset against the additional cost of the degree programme.

Introduction

Chapter 1 Key points

- The Nursing Education Forum was established by the Minister for Health and Children to prepare a strategy for the implementation of the new pre-registration nursing degree programme in 2002.

- The Forum members developed this strategy to implement the recommendations of the Commission on Nursing by adopting the principles of partnership, consultation, openness and transparency.

- This strategy aims to provide: -

  - clarity of responsibility of the stakeholders;

  - open channels of communication and consultation;

  - parity of treatment for nursing students;

  - a strategic template for change.

Background

In 1998, the Commission on Nursing presented to the Minister for Health and Children a report on the future of nursing in Ireland[1]. Following this report the Minister for Health and Children established the Nursing Education Forum[2] in February 1999. The Forum's mandate was to prepare a workable strategy to effectively and efficiently implement the recommendations made by the Commission on Nursing in relation to pre-registration nursing education in Ireland.

The Report of the Commission on Nursing advocated a change of direction in nursing education in Ireland that would ensure the continued development and progression of nursing practice and expertise in keeping with international trends and developments in best practice. This would enable Irish nurses to continue to meet the challenges of an increasingly patient-centred, results-focused, technology-driven and multi-disciplinary approach to healthcare delivery in Ireland. The Commission on Nursing also maintained that any change in educational direction must enshrine the values of caring and compassion that are integral to Irish nursing.

In brief, the key recommendations of the Commission on Nursing on pre-registration nursing education in Ireland were that:-

- pre-registration nursing education in Ireland should be a third-level four-year degree-based programme in line with international trends to enable best practice and optimise career path development for people entering the profession;
- the transition to a degree-based programme should be nationwide and should start in the academic year of 2002-2003;

- the four-year degree programme, which could lead to the awarding of an honours degree, should encompass theory and clinical practice in three nursing divisions: general, psychiatric and mental handicap.

The Establishment of a Forum on Nursing Education

The interim report of the Commission on Nursing identified concerns amongst the nursing profession with the difficulties encountered in the transition to a pre-registration nursing diploma programme between 1994 and 1998. In its final report, the Commission on Nursing recognised that the introduction of a pre-registration degree programme would require careful implementation. In particular, it identified the need for a carefully planned transition period from the pre-registration diploma programme to the pre-registration degree programme. To this end, the Commission on Nursing recommended the establishment of a Forum, with an independent chair, involving the stakeholders in education and health service provision to develop a strategic framework for the introduction of a pre-registration nursing degree programme. The Commission also recommended that the Forum examine the funding of a pre-registration degree programme.

The Minister for Health and Children established the Forum in February 1999 with the following terms of reference:-

- *to prepare a strategy for the implementation of a four-year pre-registration nursing education degree programme;*
- *to estimate the additional costs arising from the introduction of such a four-year degree programme as a replacement for the present three-year diploma programme;*

---

[1] Government of Ireland (1998) *Report of the Commission on Nursing: A Blueprint for the Future*. Dublin: Stationery Office.
[2] Throughout this report the "Nursing Education Forum" will be referred to as "the Forum".

- *to consider the respective weightings that should be given to academic achievement and general suitability in the context of the transfer of the application system for entry to pre-registration nursing education to the Central Applications Office (CAO), and to furnish recommendations to the Minister for Health and Children in relation to this matter as a matter of urgency;*
- *to consult extensively with nurse teachers involved in the development and delivery of the registration / diploma programmes;*
- *to report to the Minister for Health and Children by the 30th September, 2000.*

In carrying out its terms of reference, the Nursing Education Forum shall have regard to the relevant recommendations of the Report of the Commission on Nursing A Blueprint for the Future, and to the Final Report of the Independent External Evaluation Team, University of Southampton, on Nurse Education and Training Evaluation in Ireland.

The successful transition of nursing education to the third-level four-year degree model is dependent on a high level of ongoing partnership, communication, transparency and goodwill among and within the stakeholders in nursing education in Ireland. These include An Bord Altranais, third-level institutions, health service providers, policy makers, nurse teachers and nursing students. The stakeholder / partnership model is illustrated in Figure 1.1.

NEATE Report

The final report of the independent external evaluation team, University of Southampton, on nurse education and training evaluation in Ireland (1998)[3] - the NEATE report - identified four key

Figure 1.1:   Stakeholder / Partnership Model

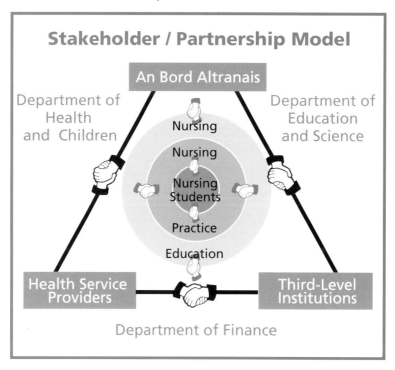

[3] Simons, H., Clarke, J.B., Gobbi, M., Long, G., Mountford, M. and Wheelhouse, C. (1998) *Nurse Education and Training Evaluation in Ireland. Independent External Evaluation. Final Report.* Southampton: University of Southampton. Hereafter referred to as the NEATE report.

factors necessary for the development and future direction of pre-registration nursing education in Ireland. These were that:-

- the theory and practice of nursing itself needs to remain the central focus of any pre-registration nursing education programme in terms of content, delivery and results;
- partnership at strategic, as well as local level, between the stakeholders in nursing education in Ireland is critical to the success of any pre-registration nursing education programme;
- control mechanisms and lines of responsibility amongst the stakeholders in nursing education in Ireland must be clearly identified and democratically agreed upon in terms of developing, implementing and evaluating a pre-registration nursing education programme;
- stakeholders in nursing education in Ireland must discuss, debate and clarify the future role of, and vision for, Irish-educated nurses in increasingly multi-disciplinary healthcare teams.

Working Principles

From the outset, and by members' agreement, the Forum adhered to four working principles in its approach to developing an effective and achievable strategy for the implementation of relevant recommendations outlined in the report of the Commission on Nursing. The four working principles were:-

Partnership

Stakeholders in nursing education in Ireland were actively represented by individual members of the Forum. In working together, members sought to model partnership approaches. Where sub committees and task groups were formed, the composition was such as to ensure that stakeholder interests relevant to the task were represented.

Consultation

Throughout its term of office, the Forum consulted with key individuals and interest groups and invited submissions from interested parties and members of the public[4]. The Forum held two consultative meetings with all nurse teachers. It also established a representative consultative sub-group of nurse teachers and held six meetings with them. Three internal briefing papers[5] and three specialist discussion papers that reviewed the extensive literature on best practice in nursing education were commissioned[6]. The Forum also built on the learning derived from the nationwide consultation exercise of the Commission on Nursing.

Openness and Transparency

Through ongoing consultative meetings, public submissions, newsletters (distributed to over 40,000 stakeholders nationwide), and a website (www.nursingeducationforum.ie, updated on a fortnightly basis), all work in progress and findings of the Forum were available to members of the public throughout its term of office. The Forum welcomed, relied on, and is grateful for all submissions, which in turn assisted the identification of key issues and the consequent development of this strategy.

---

[4] 64 submissions were received and are listed in Appendix 1.

[5] Internal briefing papers commissioned by the Forum were: Carney, M. (1999) "An Analysis of the Costing of the Registration/Diploma in Nursing in the Republic of Ireland". Dublin: School of Nursing and Midwifery, University College Dublin. Creedon, S. and Savage, E. (2000) "An Examination of Clinical Placements in Preparation for the Undergraduate BSc Nurse Education Programme scheduled to commence in 2002". Cork: Department of Nursing Studies, National University of Ireland, Cork. School of Nursing and Midwifery Studies (2000) "Evaluation and Quality Improvement". Dublin: Trinity College Dublin.

[6] The discussion papers are available from the website (www.nursingeducationforum.ie) and their titles included: Joyce, P. (2000) *Curriculum Design Principles*. Dublin: Faculty of Nursing, Royal College of Surgeons in Ireland. McCarthy, M. (2000) *Creating and Maintaining a Clinical Learning Environment*. Dublin: School of Nursing and Midwifery Studies, Trinity College Dublin. McNamara, M. (2000) *The Recruitment and Selection of Nursing Students*. Dublin: Nursing Careers Centre, An Bord Altranais.

Adherence to the spirit and letter of the Report of the Commission on Nursing in relation to pre-registration nursing education in Ireland

The Forum's remit was to develop a strategy that would enable the effective and efficient implementation of the approved relevant recommendations of the Commission on Nursing. These recommendations were developed following ongoing consultation with all the stakeholders in nursing education in Ireland. It was not within the mandate of the Forum to re-examine these recommendations.

To implement the recommendations of the Commission on Nursing on pre-registration nursing education in Ireland, the Forum decided that its strategy should:-

- clarify the lines of responsibility of all involved in pre-registration nursing education and identify the resources required for the delivery of a four-year degree programme;
- have open ongoing communication channels between the stakeholders and consultation with other expert advisers[7] integral to the successful implementation of the third-level four-year pre-registration nursing education degree programme in Ireland;
- ensure that nursing students are treated fairly and therefore subject to the same terms and conditions pertaining to other third-level students while at the same time complying with An Bord Altranais registration requirements and EU directives;
- provide a strategic template for the implementation of the degree programme rather than a detailed action plan that has potential to impair local flexibility in programme delivery.

The recommendations in this strategy for the implementation of a four-year pre-registration nursing education degree programme in Ireland, commencing in 2002, are intrinsically inter-related and interlinked and to this end the Forum suggests that they should be interpreted in their entirety.

Forum Membership

The Forum comprised thirty-four nominated representatives from various organisations actively involved in nursing education in Ireland. All members were independently appointed by the Minister for Health and Children. The independent Chair was appointed by the Minister for Health and Children, in consultation with the Minister for Education and Science.

The Forum met as a body forty-six times during its lifetime. In addition to these meetings, a number of sub committees were formed to consider and develop specific aspects of the Forum's mandate, and to report back to the Forum with their findings and recommendations. The composition of the Forum is detailed on the following pages.

[7] Expert advisers are listed in Appendix 2.

Members of the Forum

Chair:

- Dr Laraine Joyce, Deputy Director, Office for Health Management.

Members at Completion of Final Report:

- Dr Cecily Begley, Director, School of Nursing and Midwifery Studies, Trinity Centre for Health Sciences, St James's Hospital, Dublin.
- Professor Seamus Cowman, Head of Faculty of Nursing and Midwifery, Royal College of Surgeons in Ireland.
- Professor Rosemary Crow, Visiting Professor, Department of Nursing Studies, Dublin City University.
- Ms Deirdre Daly, Midwife Tutor, School of Midwifery, Rotunda Hospital, Dublin.
- Mr Ian Devlin, Administrative Officer, Department of Finance.
- Ms Mary Duff, Director of Nursing, Our Lady of Lourdes Hospital, Drogheda.
- Mr Martin Farrell, Director of Nursing, Northern Area Health Board.
- Ms Geraldine Graham, Assistant Director of Nursing, General Hospital, Portlaoise.
- Mr John Griffin, Director of Nursing, Cregg House, Sligo.
- Ms Bridget Howley, General Manager, University College Hospital, Galway.
- Ms Noreen Keane, Service Nurse Manager, Mater Misericordiae Hospital, Dublin.
- Ms Mary Kerr, Deputy Secretary, Higher Education Authority.
- Ms Josephine Leyden, Principal Nurse Tutor, James Connolly Memorial Hospital.
- Ms Emily Logan, Director of Nursing, Our Lady's Hospital for Sick Children, Crumlin.
- Dr Eric Martin, Head of School of Science, Waterford Institute of Technology.
- Mr Dermot McCarthy, Assistant Principal Officer, Department of Finance.

- Professor Geraldine McCarthy-Haslam, Head of Department of Nursing Studies, National University of Ireland, Cork.
- Dr David P Moore, Adelaide Hospital Society.
- Ms Nora Mulcahy, Director, Centre for Nursing Studies, University of Limerick.
- Mr Willie Murphy, Personnel Officer, North Western Health Board.
- Ms Honor Nicholl, Principal Nurse Tutor, The Children's Hospital, Temple Street, Dublin.
- Dr John Nolan, Registrar, National University of Ireland.
- Mr John O' Brien, Assistant Chief Executive Officer, Mid-Western Health Board.
- Ms Siobhan O'Halloran, Nursing Advisor, Nursing Policy Division, Department of Health and Children.
- Ms Sheila O'Malley, President, An Bord Altranais.
- Ms Bridget O'Neill, Principal Nurse Tutor, St Mary's, Drumcar.
- Ms Yvonne O'Shea, Chief Education Officer, An Bord Altranais.
- Dr Marian O'Sullivan, Registrar for Science and Computing, National Council for Educational Awards.
- Ms Patrice O'Sullivan, Principal Nurse Tutor, Mater Misericordiae Hospital, Dublin.
- Ms Susan Reilly, Assistant Principal Officer, Nursing Policy Division, Department of Health and Children.
- Ms Rosemary Ryan, Director of Nursing, St James's Hospital, Dublin.
- Ms Ann Sheridan, Principal Nurse Tutor, St John of God Hospital, Stillorgan.
- Mr Michael Troy, Assistant Principal Officer, Department of Education and Science.
- Ms Mary Wynne, Project Manager, Nursing, Adelaide and Meath Hospital, Dublin, incorporating The National Children's Hospital, Tallaght, Dublin.

Members of the Forum

Resignations from the Forum:

- Ms Eleanor Ní Bhriain, Principal Officer, Department of Education and Science, resigned on 9 March 1999.
- Professor Roger Watson, Head of School of Nursing, Dublin City University, resigned on 9 March 1999.
- Ms Maura Conneely, Administrative Officer, Department of Finance, resigned on 13 July 1999.
- Ms Peta Taaffe, Chief Nursing Officer, Nursing Policy Division, Department of Health and Children, resigned on 6 January 2000.
- Mrs Betty Brady, Director of Nursing Studies, Dublin City University, resigned in May 2000.

The Forum wishes to record its appreciation of their valuable input to its work.

Replacements - the following members joined the Forum:

- Mr Michael Troy, Assistant Principal Officer, Department of Education and Science, joined in March 1999.
- Mr Ian Devlin, Administrative Officer, Department of Finance, joined in September 1999.
- Ms Siobhan O'Halloran, Nurse Advisor, Nursing Policy Division, Department of Health and Children, joined in January 2000.
- Professor Rosemary Crow, Visiting Professor, Department of Nursing Studies, Dublin City University, joined in May 2000.

Secretary:

- Ms Ann Judge, Assistant Director of Nursing, The Royal Hospital Donnybrook, Dublin.

The Forum would like to acknowledge its gratitude to Ann for her dedicated support and continued commitment. Her courtesy and efficiency facilitated the Forum in completing its task.

Structure of the Report

- Following this introductory chapter, **Chapter 2** outlines the broader context which informed the Forum's work and contributed to the development of a shared vision, the guiding principles for planning and implementing the nursing degree programme and the desired outcomes.

- The recruitment and selection of nursing students and promotion of nursing as a career are considered in **Chapter 3**.

- **Chapter 4** focuses on the management of the transition from the diploma to the degree programme, the need for partnership at all levels and makes recommendations on structures to manage the change.

- The regulation and design of the curriculum for the degree programme are addressed in **Chapter 5**.

- Learning the practice of nursing as part of the curriculum is discussed in **Chapter 6**.

- **Chapter 7** provides a preliminary estimate of the additional costs involved in the move to the new degree programme.

- The report ends with a final concluding note, entitled **To Conclude...**

Context and Vision

Chapter 2

- The Forum's strategy for nursing education is informed by the World Health Organisation's European Strategy for Nursing and Midwifery Education.

- It is also informed by the publications of An Bord Altranais and its view on the role and function of the nurse.

- There must be clarity regarding the desired outcome for a pre-registration nursing degree programme.

- It is important that there is a shared vision for nursing education at both national and local level.

Introduction

The mission of nursing education is the preparation of nurses to meet the health needs of diverse populations in an ever-changing healthcare environment. There are many forces including globalisation, technology, socio-economic changes and changes in disease and treatment patterns, converging at both national and international levels, which will impact on the pursuit of this mission.

The development of the Forum's strategy and vision for nursing education in Ireland is fundamentally based on the World Health Organisation's (WHO) *Nurses and Midwives for Health, A WHO European Strategy for Nursing and Midwifery Education* (1999). It defines a nurse as *"a person who, having been formally admitted to a nursing education programme, duly recognized in the Member State in which it is located, has successfully completed the prescribed course of studies in nursing and has acquired the requisite qualifications to be registered and/or legally licensed to practice nursing"*[8].

It also considers the challenges facing the nursing profession in the context of an increasing need for well-educated nurses and midwives who are flexible, accept accountability for their work, are competent to work in multi-disciplinary and multi-sectoral contexts within hospitals and the community and who can manage constant change[9]. The multi-disciplinary working group that developed this WHO strategy acknowledged the immense cultural and socio-economic diversity across Europe and the differing stages of nursing and midwifery development within each member state.

The Forum considers this document, which aims to create the context for the development of the profession, as crucial in underpinning its strategy and vision for the future of pre-registration nursing education in Ireland.

Influences on Nursing and Midwifery Education

In formulating the WHO European Strategy, the multi-disciplinary expert group recognised that nurses and midwives would have to be educated to a high standard and have opportunities for regular continuing education. The following areas, identified as influencing and challenging nursing and midwifery education, will have significant relevance in the Irish healthcare context:-

- changing demography, whereby populations are increasingly older, more culturally diverse and different societal structures are emerging;
- the nature and pattern of health problems are changing due to disease, environmental, work and lifestyle factors;
- the understanding and evidence base of health, ill health and the impact of social circumstances are evolving;
- new knowledge is being generated in relation to disease patterns, treatment methods and technological advances;
- greater emphasis is being placed on sound theoretical knowledge and research-based practice;
- changes are occurring in the way healthcare is delivered and the importance of the patient or the healthy person at its centre, irrespective of location;
- community care provision, accessibility to services and innovation in nursing skills and practices are being increasingly emphasised;
- competition for healthcare finance and human resources is intensifying.

---

[8] World Health Organisation (1999) *Nurses and Midwives for Health, A WHO European Strategy for Nursing and Midwifery Education.* paragraph 3.2.1. Copenhagen: World Health Organisation.
[9] *Ibid.*, Foreword.

Implications for Nursing Education Programmes

It is envisaged that future Irish nursing practice will increasingly take place outside the acute hospital sector and will be delivered in a diverse range of settings. This changing environment, with its inherent growing demands for care provision, establishes a fundamental and urgent need to improve the education of nurses.

Nurses are strategically placed to provide holistic care and support the partnership between the health services and the public as care provider, decision maker, communicator, community leader and manager / co-ordinator of resources, to meet the needs of patients and communities.

Pre-registration nursing degree programmes must use innovative delivery methods and be sufficiently dynamic, flexible and responsive to accommodate these and other advances and ultimately provide the value system and basis for excellent nursing practice in the future.

The Role and Function of the Nurse

An Bord Altranais developed *The Scope of Nursing and Midwifery Practice Framework* (2000)[10] to provide guidance and support to nurses and midwives in determining their roles as healthcare professionals. In this document the definition of nursing and the role of the nurse in Ireland is based on that provided by the WHO and the International Council of Nurses and is:-

"Nursing helps individuals, families and groups to determine and achieve their physical, mental and social potential, and to do so within the challenging context of the environment in which they live and work. The nurse requires competence to develop and

perform functions that promote and maintain health and comfort as well as prevent ill health. Nursing also includes the assessment, planning and giving of care during illness and rehabilitation, and encompasses the physical, mental, spiritual and social aspects of life as they affect health, illness, disability and dying.

Nursing promotes the active involvement of the individual and his or her family, friends, social group and community, as appropriate, in all aspects of health care, thus encouraging self-reliance and self-determination while promoting a healthy environment.

Nursing is both an art and a science. It requires the understanding and application of specific knowledge and skills, and it draws on knowledge and techniques derived from the humanities and the physical, social, medical and biological sciences.

Within the total healthcare environment, nurses share with other health professionals and those in other sectors of public service the function of planning, implementation and evaluation to ensure the adequacy of the health system"[11].

Guiding Principles

In developing its shared vision of nursing education, the Forum identified the following general principles that it felt should be considered in planning any pre-registration nursing degree programme. The programme should:-

- focus on the centrality of nursing care and caring for the individual in a holistic way;
- adopt a student-centred approach to teaching and learning. The personal growth and

---

[10] An Bord Altranais (2000) *The Scope of Nursing and Midwifery Practice Framework*. Dublin: An Bord Altranais.
[11] *Ibid.*, page 3.

development of each student should be encouraged and supported throughout the programme;

- engender a culture of nursing research and promote a reflective approach to care delivery by empowering the student to examine practice within a safe environment;

- provide clear educational learning outcomes to facilitate learning and reflect the importance of clinical practice and learning through practice;

- link theory to the practice of nursing and provide the basis for professional nursing practice at the level of competence that can be further enhanced by continuing education and clinical experience;

- be grounded in educational research and developed to adopt a recognised and validated model of curriculum design and evaluation;

- recognise the role of the nurse as an equal participant within the multi-disciplinary team, through the promotion of integrated education with other healthcare professionals;

- develop assessment methods to reflect the primacy of integrating theory and practice and recognise the achievements of the student in both these settings;

- advocate that lecturers on nursing modules be nurses, ideally holding a teaching qualification, who maintain their clinical links and continue to teach both the theory and practice of nursing.

The Outcome of the Nursing Degree Programme

The Forum is of the view that students qualifying from the pre-registration nursing degree programme should be professional nurses who are safe, caring, competent decision makers, willing to accept personal and professional accountability for evidence-based practice. They should be able to promote and maintain health, as well as be able to give care during illness, rehabilitation and dying. Nurse graduates should be flexible, adaptable and reflective practitioners, integral members of the multi-disciplinary team and should adopt a life-long approach to learning.

The Development of a Shared Vision

In formulating its strategy, the Forum invested considerable time in developing and agreeing a common vision for the future pre-registration nursing degree programme in Ireland. That vision is outlined in this report. **The Forum recommends that local stakeholders involved in the delivery of each pre-registration nursing degree programme should work in partnership to develop a common shared vision for nursing education.**

Recommendation

- **The Forum recommends that local stakeholders involved in the delivery of each pre-registration nursing degree programme should work in partnership to develop a common shared vision for nursing education.**

Recruitment and Selection of Nursing Students

Chapter 3

Key points

- The advantages and disadvantages of the assessment test and the interview, in the selection of nursing students, are considered.

- The selection process must be based on the principles of transparency, impartiality and efficiency.

- The promotion of nursing as a career is a shared responsibility that requires communication, collaboration and partnership between the stakeholders in nursing education.

- Mature students represent an increasingly important cohort of nursing students.

Introduction

The successful recruitment and selection of nursing students is vital to the effective delivery of healthcare and can be carried out effectively only by health service providers and third-level academic institutions working in close partnership.

Since 1995, a number of different agencies have been responsible for the application and selection system for nursing students. Selection procedures have also changed over time and in 2001 this trend will continue. The Report of the Commission on Nursing recommended that the nursing application system transfer to the Central Applications Office (CAO) in advance of the commencement of the pre-registration nursing degree programme in 2002. Arrangements for applications through the CAO for registration / diploma programmes commencing in 2001 are now in place.

As part of its terms of reference, the Forum was asked *"to consider the respective weightings that should be given to academic achievement and general suitability in the context of the transfer of the application system for entry to pre-registration nursing education to the Central Applications Office (CAO), and to furnish recommendations to the Minister for Health and Children in relation to this matter as a matter of urgency."* The Forum members considered this matter in some detail.

Selection Mechanisms for Nursing Programmes in 2000

In 2000, the selection process for standard applicants seeking places on pre-registration nursing education programmes was as outlined in Table 3.1.

Table 3.1:   **System for Selection of Standard Nursing Applicants in 2000**

- Applications to **NURSING CAREERS CENTRE, An Bord Altranais**

- **APPLICATION FORMS** returned indicating preferences

- Candidates undertook **ASSESSMENT / BIODATA TESTS**

- **RATINGS** were given based on performance in the assessment / biodata tests

- Candidates with highest ratings were called for **INTERVIEW**

- Candidates were **RANK ORDERED** according to their performance at interview

- **LEAVING CERTIFICATE RESULTS** were then considered

- Those who attained the **MINIMUM** Leaving Certificate results were **INCLUDED**

- **OFFERS OF PLACES** were made based on ranking at interview

- Successful candidates **either ACCEPTED or REJECTED** the place

- **MEDICAL CLEARANCE** and **CHARACTER REFERENCES** were sought and considered

- If satisfactory, candidates **COMMENCED THE PROGRAMME**

The Commission on Nursing identified that the assessment / biodata tests were a necessary shortlisting mechanism given that the large number of applicants would not enable every candidate to be interviewed. In the course of its deliberations, the Forum sought evidence as to the subsequent performance of the eliminated candidates in their Leaving Certificate, but such evidence was not readily available.

In the initial stages, much of the Forum's deliberations centred on the rationale for the continued use of the interview as a selection mechanism. A number of arguments in favour of the retention as well as the abolition of the interview were debated and are summarised in Table 3.2.

Despite its reservations concerning the interview process, the Forum was required by its terms of reference to make a recommendation to the Minister on the respective weighting to be given to the interview and the Leaving Certificate under the CAO nursing application system in 2001. This implied that the interview had to be retained in line with the Commission on Nursing recommendation and the Forum accordingly recommended to the Minister in June 1999 that:

"A total of 700 points to be awarded between the Leaving Certificate and the interview i.e. up to a maximum of 600 points for the Leaving Certificate and 100 points for passing the interview. Candidates would have to meet the minimum educational requirements and pass the interview. They could be eliminated from the selection process if they failed the interview."

Since this recommendation was made, further developments have ensued with the publication

Table 3.2:   Advantages and Disadvantages of Retaining the Interview

Advantages	Disadvantages
• Long tradition of being used in the recruitment and selection of future employees	• Not a suitable selection method for a place on an educational programme
• Provides a means to screen out unsuitable candidates	• Inconsistent results and regional variations in interview panels
• The interview process allows candidates to reflect on the realities of nursing as a career	• Inefficient, costly and time consuming
• Low attrition rates	• Further compounds the health service workforce difficulties
• Report of Commission on Nursing indicated that the nursing profession might not have been ready to change	• Poor predictor of academic performance
	• Lacks transparency
	• Low reliability and validity
	• Subjective in nature with the potential for bias
	• CAO will not readily incorporate an interview after the Leaving Certificate results

of the report of the Commission on the Points System[12] and a recommendation from An Bord Altranais to the Department of Health and Children in April 2000 regarding the future selection of nursing students.

The Commission on the Points System examined the use of standardised psychometric tests as a selection tool for entry to third-level institutions. Having considered the advantages and disadvantages of both aptitude and personality assessment tests, it concluded that these methods lacked the transparency, impartiality and simplicity required of any selection mechanism. It recommended that the requisite knowledge, understanding, skills and competencies necessary should be assessed through the Leaving Certificate examination alone.

In addition, the Commission on the Points System also considered the use of interviews as a selection tool for entry to third-level programmes and felt that their subjective nature could lead to bias in selection. Evidence also suggested that they were a poor predictor of academic performance. The organisational effort involved and the resource implications in terms of training, time, travel, and cost were difficult to justify in light of the concerns regarding the validity and reliability of interviews. It recommended therefore that interviews should not be used as a selection method for standard applicants entering third-level educational programmes.

The recommendations of the Commission on the Points System have yet to be approved by Government. However, in April 2000, An Bord Altranais recommended to the Department of Health and Children that both the written assessment test and interview be discontinued for school leaver applicants under the CAO Nursing

Application System from 2001. It also recommended that the selection of school leavers for nursing should be based solely on points obtained in the Leaving Certificate examination. The Forum endorsed the recommendation of An Bord Altranais when the Department of Health and Children sought its views on this issue in May 2000.

The Forum believes that there should be parity of treatment between applicants to nursing programmes and applicants to other third-level courses. The selection process should be based on the principles of transparency, impartiality and efficiency and must be capable of securing the support of both the profession and the general public. **The Forum recommends that the assessment test and the interview for school leavers be discontinued from 2001 under the transfer of the application system to the CAO.**

Selection Mechanisms for Nursing Programmes in 2001

As recommended in the Report of the Commission on Nursing, the administration of the selection process has been transferred to the CAO for 2001, in advance of the move to the degree programme. Standard applicants applying for pre-registration nursing education programmes will be competing on the basis of Leaving Certificate points only.

The standard system operated by the CAO gives applicants two sets of choices, one for degree courses and another for diploma / certificate courses. Up to ten courses may be chosen in each set. In 2001, the addition of the Nursing Applications System will give applicants a third set of choices for nursing courses.

---

[12] Government of Ireland (1999) *Commission on the Points System: Final Report and Recommendations.* Dublin: Stationery Office.

To this end, a separate application form and nursing application handbook have been devised and are now available from the CAO. The form contains three nursing lists and applicants will be able to select from up to ten general, ten psychiatric and eight mental handicap nursing education programmes.

The Commission on the Points System was not in favour of an increase in the number of lists available on the CAO form. Whilst it acknowledged the special circumstances relating to nursing, it identified this as an issue for further consideration. **The Forum recommends that An Bord Altranais monitor and review on a continuing basis the issue of the separate CAO lists for nursing.**

Promotion and Marketing of Nursing as a Career

The promotion and marketing of nursing as a career is a shared responsibility that requires partnership and collaboration between the stakeholders.

The changes in the application and selection system, particularly over the past five years, have led to a degree of confusion among potential applicants, their parents and teachers. This perceived lack of clarity needs to be addressed by means of a co-ordinated and appropriately targeted promotional and marketing campaign which will ensure that the number of applicants is maintained at a high level.

Good practice in the recruitment of students to nursing degree programmes includes:-

- the production and dissemination of high-quality promotional materials;
- the development of internet websites;

- effective liaison with health service providers and nurse educators;
- networking with schools and community resource centres;
- effective communication with guidance counsellors at local and national level;
- participation in local, national and international careers conferences;
- the development and implementation of local and national media strategies;
- the establishment of a network of nurses involved in the promotion of nursing.

The Forum recommends that An Bord Altranais continue to co-ordinate and provide strategic direction to the promotion and marketing of nursing as a career.

Recent Trends in Nursing Applications

The first preference of an applicant is one index of strength of preference for a particular discipline of nursing. The Forum examined the distribution of first preferences of applicants to nursing in 1999 and 2000, supplied by An Bord Altranais. There is tentative evidence to suggest that requiring applicants to commit to undertake a specific discipline of nursing at the point of access may have an adverse effect on recruitment to psychiatric and mental handicap nursing. In order to explore this evidence in greater detail **the Forum recommends that An Bord Altranais undertake further research to examine the rationale for, and impact of, maintaining three points of access to pre-registration nursing.** This is required as part of an overall review of factors impacting on recruitment into nursing.

The Commission on Nursing considered that the current non-means tested grant to nursing students may not be tenable when pre-registration nursing education becomes incorporated into the third-level education sector. On the principle of equality of treatment with other third-level students this grant will no longer be payable in 2002 and nursing students will be means tested for grants in the future. **The Forum recommends that An Bord Altranais monitor the impact of the withdrawal of the non-means tested grant.**

Sick Children's Nursing

The Commission on Nursing indicated that the qualification in sick children's nursing should remain a post-registration qualification. Concern was raised in the submissions to the Forum and in discussions with nurse teachers that sick children's nursing was not being offered at pre-registration level. The Forum noted the issue but considered that it fell outside its terms of reference. The Forum also noted that a working group had been established by the Department of Health and Children to review the provision of sick children's nursing education.

The Adelaide Hospital Society

The Commission on Nursing identified that the recruitment and selection of nursing students for the Adelaide Hospital Society in the future was an issue for discussion and negotiation between the Adelaide Hospital Society and the CAO. These discussions have concluded and the CAO has put arrangements in place for 2001 for both standard and mature applicants to the Adelaide School of Nursing, Trinity College Dublin.

Mature Students

Mature applicants represent an increasingly significant proportion of those applying to nursing education programmes[13]. Demographic

trends indicate that the number of school leavers is expected to drop in the future.

The Commission on Nursing recommended that a bursary / sponsorship system be put in place by the Department of Health and Children to promote applications to all divisions by mature applicants. In light of the recent trends in relation to mature nursing applicants **the Forum recommends that discussions on the framework for a bursary / sponsorship system for mature nursing students commence as soon as possible between the Department of Health and Children, An Bord Altranais and health service providers.**

In addition, the Commission on Nursing recommended that a quota of places for mature students be established in each third-level institution providing pre-registration nursing education programmes[14].

The Commission on the Points System recommended that a comprehensive guidance counselling and information service be provided for mature students and that third-level institutions bear in mind their specific needs in the preparation and provision of information for prospective students. It also distinguished between the selection criteria appropriate for standard applicants and those that might be used for mature applicants and recommended that a single evaluation of a mature person's application under a co-ordinated system of assessment should be established by the CAO for the 2002 intake[15].

Given that mature entrants may increasingly form a significant proportion of students on nursing education programmes, consideration must be

---

[13] The proportion of mature applicants for nursing education programmes rose from 14% in 1997 to 29% in 2000.

[14] A quota of places has already been established in each third-level institution following a consultation exercise early in 2000 and it will be subject to refinement depending on the outcome of the process in 2001.

[15] A single co-ordinated system of assessment for mature nursing applicants under the CAO, involving interviews and aptitude tests, has been established for 2001. Discussions are ongoing regarding subsequent selection mechanisms.

given to their specific learning and developmental needs. Mechanisms need to be put in place to evaluate each individual applicant's suitability for the clinical, as well as the academic demands of the programme. The Forum recommends that third-level institutions and health service providers make provision for the support that mature students will require to under-take the pre-registration nursing degree programme.

Recommendations

- The Forum recommends that the assessment test and the interview for school leavers be discontinued from 2001 under the transfer of the application system to the CAO.
- The Forum recommends that An Bord Altranais monitor and review on a continuing basis the issue of the separate CAO lists for nursing.
- The Forum recommends that An Bord Altranais continue to co-ordinate and provide strategic direction to the promotion and marketing of nursing as a career.
- The Forum recommends that An Bord Altranais undertake further research to examine the rationale for, and impact of, maintaining three points of access to pre-registration nursing.
- The Forum recommends that An Bord Altranais monitor the impact of the withdrawal of the non-means tested grant.
- The Forum recommends that discussions on the framework for a bursary / sponsorship system for mature nursing students commence as soon as possible between the Department of Health and Children, An Bord Altranais and health service providers.

- The Forum recommends that third-level institutions and health service providers make provision for the support that mature students will require to undertake the pre-registration nursing degree programme.

Managing the Change

Chapter 4 Key points

- The transition to the pre-registration degree programme must be actively managed to ensure that all stakeholders are fully informed and committed to the change.

- The roles and responsibilities of the major stakeholders must be clear.

- Implementation structures are needed to move the implementation process forward.

- A communications strategy is necessary to ensure all stakeholders are informed of and can inform the change process.

Introduction

The transition to a degree-based model of nurse education will involve considerable change in the manner in which nurse education programmes are managed and delivered and the way in which clinical placements are scheduled and monitored. These, together with the transfer of staff including teachers from the health service to third-level institutions, pose challenges that require proactive management.

To be successful, close partnership is required between all stakeholders at all stages of the transition process. Moreover, the transition process must be continually monitored at national and local levels so that any existing and emerging problems can be promptly identified and properly addressed.

The Management of Change

Change of any kind involves a move away from the *status quo* and will always prompt reactions that can be both positive and negative. The key to the successful introduction and adoption of change is ongoing and open communication and consultation among all stakeholders. A degree of flexibility needs to be built into proposals so that consensus can be achieved and change effectively implemented.

The genuine commitment of all stakeholders is essential. This chapter will address the following issues and concerns that arise in managing a major change of this nature:-

- organisational and individual roles must be agreed and made explicit to all stakeholders to ensure accountability for pre-determined aspects of the programme;
- structures must be established to support the change process and its end result;

- the rationale for the proposed change must be communicated to all parties so that individual and organisational concerns can be addressed;
- other transition issues, such as implementation timescales, the development of capital infrastructure, the transfer of nurse teachers into third-level institutions and the overlap between the diploma programme and the degree programme must be addressed.

The Need for Partnership

Partnership amongst stakeholders is critical to the success of the programme and must occur at all levels. In becoming competent, safe and effective in providing patient care, nursing students need considerable exposure to clinical practice during their educational programme. Partnership between educational institutions and health service providers is therefore of vital importance. As an outcome of the programme, health service providers need competent practitioners and the third-level institutions require clinical sites providing diverse clinical learning opportunities for students. In addition, the programme must meet the professional standards specified by An Bord Altranais which in turn must reflect the needs of the health service. The full integration of nursing education into third-level institutions also requires partnership between the policy makers in the Higher Education Authority, the Department of Health and Children, the Department of Education and Science and the Department of Finance.

Principles of Effective Partnership

Partnerships require work; they do not just happen. This must be recognised by all stakeholders from the outset. Mutual respect needs to be established as well as a clear understanding of the areas of authority and competence, and the consequent roles and responsibilities of each. A framework for progression must be developed.

Based in part on the recommendations of the NEATE Report, at a central level this requires that:-

- stakeholders jointly develop and agree a shared philosophy and strategy for nursing education;
- stakeholders recognise, appreciate and work within the bounds of existing legislation regarding the regulatory, academic, clinical, professional and registration aspects of the pre-registration education of nurses;
- regulatory bodies enable curriculum development and innovation whilst safeguarding professional and academic standards;
- in planning for the future of nursing education there is wide consultation and sufficient flexibility to enable local institutions to respond flexibly to local need;
- there is clarity regarding the roles and responsibilities of each of the partners both locally and nationally.

At local level a framework for partnership requires:-

- joint structures and clear accountability;
- recognition of each partner's contribution to the programme;
- regular review and evaluation of the partnership arrangements.

The Forum recommends that, before 2002, a memorandum of understanding[16] be drawn up and signed by stakeholders at local level between each third-level institution and its related health service providers. The purpose of this is to establish a collaborative framework for the provision of the degree programme, in the spirit of the recommendations of the Commission on Nursing. The memorandum of understanding should address the following:-

- general context;
- legislative framework;

- partnership arrangements;
- co-operative structures;
- joint working group;
- student health and security screening;
- registration;
- programme content;
- clinical placements;
- assessment methodologies and examinations;
- academic approval / accreditation;
- student welfare and code of conduct;
- joint appointments;
- review;
- notice to terminate the agreement.

Responsibilities of Stakeholders

The Forum in its deliberations was conscious of the need for clarity in relation to the roles and responsibilities of the stakeholders involved in the delivery of a pre-registration nursing degree programme. Effective delivery of the programme requires good working relationships between the stakeholders and recognition of common aims whilst acknowledging the different roles and responsibilities of each partner.

The provision of a pre-registration nursing degree will involve three stakeholders: the regulatory / professional body, third-level educational institutions and health service providers. Each stakeholder has distinct responsibilities in the delivery of a degree programme. The Forum discussed these at some length. As clarity is crucial, the main responsibilities of each stakeholder are outlined below.

An Bord Altranais

The primary statutory responsibility of the regulatory / professional body - An Bord Altranais - as provided for in the Nurses Act 1985, *"is to promote high standards of professional education and training and professional conduct amongst nurses"*[17].

---

[16] Appendix 3 contains a sample of a possible memorandum of understanding. This should be adapted to reflect local circumstances.
[17] Nurses Act 1985. part 2. paragraph 6 (1).

Therefore, the primary responsibility of An Bord Altranais in relation to the pre-registration nursing degree programme is to ensure the establishment and maintenance of and adherence to professional standards in all courses preparing students for registration. The discharge of this responsibility requires An Bord Altranais to:-

- establish requirements and standards for pre-registration nurse education and training;
- ensure that all the statutory requirements of An Bord Altranais and EU Directives with respect to nurse education and training are met;
- establish minimum entry requirements for nurse education and training programmes;
- be satisfied that those presenting for registration have completed a programme of education and training in accordance with requirements and standards laid down by the Board.

Third-level Institution

The primary responsibility of the third-level institution, in relation to the pre-registration degree programme, is the education of students to degree standard in accordance with the institution's academic procedures and statutory requirements and consistent with professional registration as a nurse. Such responsibility will require the third-level institution to:-

- develop educational programmes in collaboration with health service providers;
- ensure the effective management and delivery of the degree programme;
- meet the requirements of An Bord Altranais with regard to programme validation;
- review the programme on a regular basis in accordance with quality assurance standards.

The maintenance of high academic standards

places a responsibility on third-level institutions to ensure appropriate structures and resources are in place for the effective management and delivery of the programme. The Commission on Nursing recommended the establishment of a faculty or department of nursing within each third-level institution providing a pre-registration degree programme and suggested that professors or deans of nursing should head this faculty / department and have an adequate number of lectureships in nursing to support the programme. In addition, the WHO European Strategy for Nursing and Midwifery Education suggested that the *"Director/Head of the Nursing School/Department must be a qualified nurse…"*[18]. **The Forum recommends therefore that appropriate academic structures for a nursing degree programme be established within each third-level institution such as a faculty, school or department of nursing. A nurse at an appropriate grade consistent with other academic departments should head this faculty, school or department of nursing.**

The third-level institution also has a key role in supporting students in the clinical learning environment, an integral component of the four-year degree programme.

Health Service Provider

A critical element that differentiates a pre-registration nursing degree programme from many other academic programmes is the level of clinical practice exposure in the programme. The primary responsibility of the health service provider, through the appropriate director of nursing, is to ensure the effectiveness of the clinical learning environment for the acquisition of clinical knowledge and skills. The director of nursing will be responsible for:-

[18] World Health Organisation (1999) *Nurses and Midwives for Health, A WHO European Strategy for Nursing and Midwifery Education.* paragraph 4.20. Copenhagen: World Health Organisation.

- providing an agreed number of clinical placements (both supernumerary and rostered clinical placements);
- the adequacy of such placements;
- optimising the capacity of clinical placements;
- providing effective support structures for students in the clinical environment.

Partnership and Joint Responsibility for Clinical Placements

The main area in which health service providers and third-level institutions must work closely in partnership is in relation to clinical placements. This is discussed in more detail in Chapter 6, but briefly, they are jointly responsible for:-

- maintaining effective partnership structures to support academic and clinical aspects of the programme;
- providing adequate support to clinical staff in developing and maintaining an effective learning environment;
- making adequate arrangements for clinical assessments.

Structures to Manage the Change

Because of established cultures, beliefs and values, institutional change is one of the most challenging aspects of change management. For it to happen, change must work its way through the system. To facilitate the change to a degree-based programme, those involved in the transition process must consider and understand the existing structures within Irish healthcare, third-level institutions and related organisations. The most effective means of managing change is by establishing collaborative structures that give concrete expression to partnership and ensure a formal and networked monitoring, evaluation and feedback system.

Formal structures should be put in place to facilitate networks of communication and evaluation at all levels. This in turn will inform any adaptations to the transition strategy required along the way. In addition, formal monitoring structures will enable stakeholders to forecast, plan and manage the demands made on their resources during the transition process. The structures include a national implementation committee, an inter-departmental steering committee, local joint working groups on nursing education and local project managers. The relationships between these implementation structures are outlined in Figure 4.1.

National Implementation Committee

The Forum recommends the establishment of a national implementation committee to oversee the implementation of the pre-registration nursing degree programme. It is envisaged that this will be a temporary structure to facilitate the implementation process. Where necessary, the national implementation committee would refer matters for clarification to other bodies such as the Department of Health and Children or the Department of Education and Science or the inter-departmental steering committee recommended below.

The national implementation committee membership should represent the relevant stakeholders in nursing education including An Bord Altranais, the Department of Health and Children, the Department of Education and Science, the Department of Finance, third-level institutions and health service providers. Its functions would include:-

- monitoring progress in the implementation of the pre-registration nursing degree programme across the country;

- communicating and liaising with the inter-departmental steering committee;
- receiving information from and providing advice to local joint working groups on nursing education;
- ensuring a partnership approach is adopted at a national level which will influence and inform the approach taken locally;
- communicating key developments and progress made to the public.

Communication from the national implementation committee will include the production and distribution of an annual report charting the progress of the implementation process, the commissioning of research, position or discussion papers as are deemed necessary and the provision of a website providing up-to-date information on progress and developments nationally.

The national implementation committee will

perform a vital function in overseeing this major change initiative. **The Forum recommends that the national implementation committee should be established as soon as possible and funded by the Department of Health and Children. Its initial task should be to prepare a plan of the processes and actions necessary to ensure the implementation of the Forum's recommendations in a structured, co-ordinated and coherent manner in compliance with the timescale set out in this report. The Forum recommends that the Minister for Health and Children, following consultation with the Minister for Education and Science, appoint an independent chair and the members of the national implementation committee.**

Inter-Departmental Steering Committee
The Commission on Nursing recommended that funding for the degree in nursing should remain

Figure 4.1:   Implementation Structures

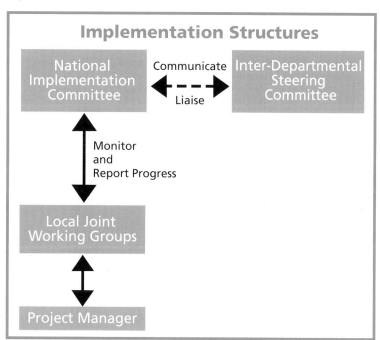

with the Department of Health and Children and become the responsibility of the Department of Education and Science once nursing education is integrated into the third-level sector. As a consequence, policy decisions concerning the nursing degree programme will continue to be made during the transition phase by the Minister for Health and Children. This will necessarily involve close consultation and collaboration with the Departments of Education and Science and Finance and with the Higher Education Authority to ensure continuity once responsibility for the nursing degree programme transfers to the Department of Education and Science.

The Forum recommends that an inter-departmental steering committee should be established to co-ordinate the activities and policies of the Departments of Health and Children and Education and Science during the transition to a degree programme. All policy and funding issues associated with the introduction of the degree programme should be considered by the inter-departmental steering committee. **The Forum recommends that the inter-departmental steering committee should comprise representatives of the Departments of Health and Children, Education and Science, Finance and the Higher Education Authority.**

The inter-departmental steering committee should liaise closely with the national implementation committee and consider any inter-departmental policy issues that may be referred to it.

Local Joint Working Groups on Nursing Education

The Forum recommends that local joint working groups on nursing education be established comprising representatives of a third-level educational institution providing pre-registration nursing education and its associated health service providers. Their purpose would be to provide a strategic overview of the change process, monitor progress and address partnership issues as may arise. The local joint working groups would normally be centred around a third-level institution and its associated health service providers. Such groups may already be in existence in some areas and can assume the functions outlined. In certain circumstances, third-level institutions might wish to collaborate with others in a geographic area and establish a regional joint working group.

The local joint working groups should be decision-making groups that are focused on providing direction and clarification on local matters pertaining to the transition to the pre-registration nursing degree programme. They would refer matters to the national implementation committee, where appropriate. Their main functions would be to:-

- monitor the progress of the transition to the degree programme through feedback from local project managers, and report progress and issues to the national implementation committee;
- monitor and advise on the process of staff preparation for the change;
- develop, implement and review a local communication strategy;
- delegate operational issues to other relevant sub committees and receive reports as appropriate;
- monitor and advise on curriculum development, implementation and evaluation.

Whilst the initial primary task of the local joint working groups is to plan for and oversee the transition to the degree programme, **the Forum recommends that the local joint working-groups on nursing education should remain in existence after the transition is complete.** This will ensure that formal structures for partnership at a local level are maintained.

Membership of these working groups should comprise relevant academic staff and individuals with designated responsibility for leading the transition process in each of the main health service providers in the area. Sub committees may be formed as required to deal with topics such as student welfare, capital development, curriculum design and evaluation and so on.

The submissions received by the Forum and consultations with nurse teachers in schools of nursing and third-level institutions, indicated the need for staff to be adequately prepared for this change. It is important therefore that induction programmes for staff within the third-level sector are established. Nurse teachers who transfer into third-level institutions may require orientation, mentoring and development in new roles. New nurse lecturers may require support and development in areas such as research, publications, academic processes and procedures. Other non-nursing academic staff associated with the programme will require orientation in terms of the educational requirements and standards of the pre-registration nursing degree programme. **The Forum recommends that formal induction programmes be provided by the third-level institutions to facilitate the transfer and integration of nurse teachers into the third-level sector.**

The health service providers will have responsibility for ensuring that their nursing staff are adequately prepared for the change. This issue is considered in Chapter 6.

Local Project Managers

The transition to the degree programme will entail complex changes for all stakeholders and these changes must be managed. For this to happen responsibility for managing the change at local level must be devolved to designated individuals. **The Forum recommends that one individual should be designated as project manager of the transition to the degree programme for the duration of the transition process by each local joint working group on nursing education.**

This position should have sufficient time allocated to it, and not be given as an additional responsibility to an existing full-time role. However, it may not necessarily be a full-time post in itself. The appointee should command the respect and trust of managers and staff, and be skilled as a facilitator. The project manager should be a member of the local joint working group and report progress regularly to it. The key responsibilities of a project manager are to:-

- facilitate and co-ordinate the change process at an operational level within the constituent organisations;
- support the existing nursing student population by clearly communicating the implications of the degree-based programme to them, and by providing an interactive platform for student discussion and feedback;
- explain the process of transition to the degree programme to staff within the organisations;
- ensure relevant staff are prepared for the new degree programme;
- monitor and evaluate the progress of the transition process continually, and report relevant issues to the local joint working group.

Communications Strategy

At each level of implementation there is a responsibility to communicate on developments in nursing education to relevant stakeholders, as indicated in Table 4.1. **The Forum recommends that the national implementation committee, inter-departmental steering committee and local joint working groups should each draw up and implement a strategy for communication with their relevant stakeholders and each other.** The purpose of the communication strategy at these levels should be to ensure that those who will be affected by the proposed changes are fully briefed on the reasons for the change and have an opportunity to discuss their possible implications.

Transition Issues

Transfer of Nurse Teachers

The recommendations of the Commission on Nursing on the transition to a four-year degree-based programme of pre-registration nursing education have implications for the future career paths of existing nurse teachers. The conditions under which nurse teachers will transfer to the third-level institutions are the subject of ongoing discussions between the Department of Health and Children, the Department of Education and Science, the Health Service Employers Agency, the Higher Education Authority, the nursing unions and representatives of third-level institutions involved in the provision of pre-registration nursing education. The successful conclusion of these discussions will facilitate the transition

Table 4.1:   **Communications Framework**

Level	Stakeholder	Action
• National implementation committee	• The general public • Professional groups	• Periodic public statements • Publication of annual report • Website • Circulation of bi-annual newsletter • Research, discussion and position papers
• Inter-departmental steering committee	• Relevant stakeholders	• Ministerial statements, speeches and policy documents
• Local joint working groups	• Relevant staff in organisations represented • Students	• Annual report and periodic progress reports to national implementation committee • Newsletter / bulletin to brief on ongoing developments • Policy documents

process. The Forum recognises the central role that nurse teachers will continue to play in the provision of pre-registration nursing education.

Implementation Timescale

Subject to the acceptance of this report by the Minster for Health and Children, the timescale for the implementation of the transfer of nursing education into third-level is indicated in Table 4.2. The timescale is demanding on all stakeholders and assumes that:-

- a Government decision to proceed with implementation is taken by the end of 2000;
- all third-level institutions will have their programmes ready for validation by February 2001;
- appropriate accommodation and other resource requirements for students are identified and made available.

Table 4.2:   Implementation Timescale

October 2000	**Nursing Education Forum reports to Minister for Health and Children.**
November 2000 - December 2000	**Inter-departmental steering committee on integration of nursing students within third-level.** The inter-departmental steering committee considers the student, staff and accommodation requirements for the integration of nursing students within third-level institutions. **Local joint working groups on nursing education.** Established to plan for and oversee the transition to the degree programme.
January 2001	**National implementation committee is established by the Minister for Health and Children in consultation with the Minister for Education and Science.**
February 2001	**Validation of new degree programme completed.** The validation process for all new four-year degree programmes in nursing at third-level to be completed.
March 2001	**CAO list for 2002 / 2003 is finalised.**
June 2001	**CAO list is printed.**
1 February 2002	**Closing date for CAO applications.**
August 2002	**CAO offer of a place in new four-year degree programme.** The Leaving Certificate results to be issued and places offered to students in the new four-year degree programme in nursing.
September 2002	**New four-year degree programme in nursing commences.** The first cohort of students register for, and commence their courses of study in the new four-year degree programme at third-level.

Capital Development

The estimated costs of the necessary capital development required in the third-level sector to accommodate the increased number of nursing students on third-level campuses are indicated in Chapter 7. The development of physical facilities within third-level institutions will require careful planning. There is, in general, a timescale of three years from the decision to commence with a particular project to the completion of the building programme. However, prior to the decision to accept any proposal for capital development, careful evaluation by the relevant department with responsibility for the capital project would be required. A capital investment of the size which may be required to integrate nursing students onto third-level campuses will require careful consideration and evaluation by the Departments of Health and Children, Education and Science and Finance.

The Commission on Nursing recommended that nursing students be integrated within the general third-level student body. However, it is recognised that the scale of capital investment required to facilitate physical integration is such that a phased capital investment programme will be required. **The Forum recommends that the inter-departmental steering committee undertake, as a matter of priority, a detailed analysis for each third-level institution, of the necessary capital investment required. In addition, the Forum recommends that every reasonable effort be made to facilitate the full physical integration of nursing students within third-level institutions at the earliest practicable date.**

Service Implications

The implementation of the changes will have implications for health service providers. The key issue facing nurse managers is one of ensuring a consistently high quality of care whilst at the same time facilitating student learning. Students on the rostered placement will be paid employees of health service providers but will still require support and supervision in practice. The replacement of nurses with rostered students has implications for the skill mix within the service.

In addition, the current shortage of nursing personnel and the increased ratio of support staff may reduce the ratio of nurses to students and consequently dictate the number of students that can be accommodated in any one area. These factors will have to be considered when replacement ratios are calculated at local level.

The Overlap between the Diploma and Degree Programmes

The Commission on Nursing recommended that the degree programme should commence in all relevant third-level institutions on a national basis at the start of the academic year in 2002. The final cohort of diploma students will complete their programme in 2004. There will thus be an overlap of two years during which students undertaking the diploma are completing their programme and the new students are starting their degree programme. This issue was discussed with nurse teachers and it was generally agreed that it would be preferable for all nursing students and nurse teachers, who wish to transfer, to integrate into third-level institutions at the same time. **The Forum recommends that all nursing students, both diploma and degree, and those nurse teachers who wish to move into third-level should be fully integrated into the third-level system in time for the start of the degree programme in 2002.**

It was suggested that integration might take place as early as possible to facilitate joint planning and programme development. The Forum considers that it should be up to each third-level institution and its associated schools of nursing to decide when full integration should take place. This may vary depending on local circumstances. In addition, it is important that the needs of students undertaking the diploma programme are not overlooked in this process. They should benefit also from the integration into third-level and it should be carefully managed to minimise any disruption to their programme.

Recommendations

- The Forum recommends that, before 2002, a memorandum of understanding be drawn up and signed by stakeholders at local level between each third-level institution and its related health service providers.
- The Forum recommends that appropriate academic structures for a nursing degree programme be established within each third-level institution such as a faculty, school or department of nursing. A nurse at an appropriate grade consistent with other academic departments should head this faculty, school or department of nursing.
- The Forum recommends the establishment of a national implementation committee to oversee the implementation of the pre-registration nursing degree programme.
- The Forum recommends that the national implementation committee should be established as soon as possible and funded by the Department of Health and Children. Its initial task should be to prepare a plan of the processes and actions necessary to

ensure the implementation of the Forum's recommendations in a structured, co-ordinated and coherent manner in compliance with the timescale set out in this report. The Forum recommends that the Minister for Health and Children, following consultation with the Minister for Education and Science, appoint an independent chair and the members of the national implementation committee.

- The Forum recommends that an inter-departmental steering committee should be established to co-ordinate the activities and policies of the Departments of Health and Children and Education and Science during the transition to a degree programme.
- The Forum recommends that the inter-departmental steering committee should comprise representatives of the Departments of Health and Children, Education and Science, Finance and the Higher Education Authority.
- The Forum recommends that local joint working groups on nursing education be established comprising representatives of a third-level educational institution providing pre-registration nursing education and its associated health service providers.
- The Forum recommends that the local joint working groups on nursing education should remain in existence after the transition is complete.
- The Forum recommends that formal induction programmes be provided by the third-level institutions to facilitate the transfer and integration of nurse teachers into the third-level sector.
- The Forum recommends that one individual should be designated as project

manager of the transition to the degree programme for the duration of the transition process by each local joint working group on nursing education.

- The Forum recommends that the national implementation committee, inter-departmental steering committee and local joint working groups should each draw up and implement a strategy for communication with their relevant stakeholders and each other.

- The Forum recommends that the inter-departmental steering committee undertake, as a matter of priority, a detailed analysis for each third-level institution, of the necessary capital investment required. In addition, the Forum recommends that every reasonable effort be made to facilitate the full physical integration of nursing students within third-level institutions at the earliest practicable date.

- The Forum recommends that all nursing students, both diploma and degree, and those nurse teachers who wish to move into third-level should be fully integrated into the third-level system in time for the start of the degree programme in 2002.

The Curriculum - Regulation and Design

Chapter 5   Key points

- Curriculum design for pre-registration nursing education must take place within the regulatory framework of An Bord Altranais requirements and standards and EU Directives.

- Principles to guide curriculum design will provide a common focus whilst permitting local flexibility.

- All relevant stakeholders need to be involved in curriculum design, delivery and evaluation.

Introduction

The regulatory framework for nursing, and the principles that the Forum considers should inform curriculum design in preparing for the nursing degree programme, are outlined in this chapter. The Nurse Education and Training Evaluation in Ireland - the NEATE Report - identified that the curriculum for the diploma programme was centrally imposed and as a result there was insufficient flexibility to allow adaptation to local needs. The Forum considers that the principles contained in this chapter can act as a guide to curriculum design which can be interpreted locally. The use of principles to guide curriculum development serves to provide a common focus without being too prescriptive. In this respect, the approach has the potential to accommodate local interpretation for the process of curriculum design. It is important that the curriculum is developed in partnership between third-level institutions and local health service providers. However, a curriculum must be designed in the context of the national statutory framework for nursing education and relevant EU Directives on nursing education.

Statutory Framework for Nursing Education

Programmes of study and qualifications in nursing education at third-level are governed by certain provisions in the Universities Act (1997), the NCEA Act (1979), the Regional Technical Colleges Acts (1992 and 1999) and the Qualifications (Education and Training) Act (1999)[19].

The Nurses Rules, 1988 (Amendment) Rules, 1998 and 1999 in accordance with the Nurses Act (1985) make provision for third-level institutions and healthcare institutions to develop curricula based on An Bord Altranais' *Requirements and Standards for Nurse Registration Education Programmes* (1999). This document aspires to *"provide guidance for the development of flexible, innovative, practice-oriented registration programmes to third-level institutions and health care institutions involved in the education and training of nurses"*[20].

The criteria established by An Bord Altranais must fulfill the appropriate EU Directives on general nursing and midwifery, European Community Directives. In 1989, a directive from the Council of European Communities (89/595/EEC) stated that the length of theoretical instruction should be at least one-third, and that of clinical instruction at least one-half, of the minimum length of training, which is 4,600 hours[21].

With this in mind, the Forum needed to ensure that the essential components of the degree programme, as specified by the EU, could be facilitated in the four-year programme as envisaged by the Commission on Nursing. Accordingly, a study to examine how all the requirements could be met in practice was commissioned[22]. This study concluded that the requirements were achievable within the four-year period while at the same time ensuring that nursing students had equity with other third-level students' vacations during all parts of the programme, with the exception of the rostered year.

---

[19] The Qualifications (Education and Training) Act (1999) which has been passed by the Oireachtas, will come into effect when the Minister for Education and Science signs the commencement order.

[20] An Bord Altranais (1999) *Requirements and Standards for Nurse Registration Education Programmes*. page 5. Dublin: An Bord Altranais.

[21] Council of European Communities (1989) "Council Directive (89/595/EEC)", *Official Journal of the European Communities*, L 341, Vol.32, 23 November 1989.

[22] Creedon, S. and Savage, E. (2000) "An Examination of Clinical Placements in Preparation for the Undergraduate BSc Nurse Education Programme scheduled to commence in 2002". Cork: Department of Nursing Studies, National University of Ireland, Cork.

The NEATE Report Findings in Relation to the Curriculum

The Forum was cognisant of the NEATE Report findings on the Galway diploma programme which highlighted that:-

- the curriculum design was adversely affected by the regulatory frameworks of An Bord Altranais and the University;
- disagreements arose about the scheduling of subjects and clinical placements throughout the programme;
- there were differences of opinion concerning the nature, purpose and scheduling of tuition in the biological and social sciences;
- students experienced an intensive, theoretically overloaded and overassessed curriculum during the first thirty-six weeks of the programme;
- the separate assessment of theory and clinical practice was creating a theory-practice gap, exacerbated by the emphasis on theory and the neglect of clinical experience in the early part of the programme.

These issues indicate the need for a partnership approach to curriculum design and delivery and the NEATE Report recommended that all the stakeholders in nursing education should have a clear and shared long-term vision for nursing and nursing education in Ireland.

Curriculum Models

Three potential models of professional nursing education were outlined in the NEATE Report. These were:-

- pre-technocratic model;
- technocratic model;
- post-technocratic model.

The **pre-technocratic** or apprenticeship model represents professional education that takes place largely "on the job" with some instruction given through block and / or day release in an associated training school or institute of higher education. Curriculum content and assessment strategies focus on the learning and acquisition of practical routines and the knowledge necessary to both acquire and practise these routines.

The **technocratic** model is characterised by the location of student learning in schools associated with third-level education. Academic subject specialists often deliver curriculum content. Knowledge is interpreted and applied to practice.

In the **post-technocratic** model emphasis is placed on the acquisition of professional competencies that are primarily developed through experience of, and reflection on practice, in a practice setting where students have access to a skilled practitioner. This setting can be located in the employing agency or academic institution or in both. It is envisaged that such an arrangement will provide a link between the academic institution and the world of practice and between professional education and subsequent employment. The curriculum based on the post-technocratic model promotes the development of reflection on practice and the acquisition of skills to use reflection, observation, analysis and evaluation to develop nursing practices.

The Forum recommends that discussion on the model of professional education to underpin the nursing degree programme should take place between third-level institutions and health service providers. The purpose of this is to ensure that there is a common shared vision of the underlying model of professional education that is being adopted.

The Forum, based on its consultations and investigations, suggests that a post-technocratic model, with elements of the technocratic model, is the appropriate model for pre-registration nursing education.

Core Principles to Guide Curriculum Design

The use of core principles provides curricular direction while allowing for adaptation to meet particular needs in individual curricula. From its consultations and discussions, the Forum identified the core principles of flexibility, eclecticism, transferability and progression, utility, evidence base and shared learning to guide curriculum design and suggests that these should underpin curriculum development.

Flexibility

This principle refers to the need for autonomy to design curricula in a manner that is responsive to local needs. A number of different models of professional education and curriculum were proposed in submissions made to the Forum. These included the spiral model, the fourfold curriculum model, and the post-technocratic model of professional education. Regardless of the curriculum model chosen **the Forum recommends that the curriculum design be dynamic and flexible to permit responsiveness to local needs.**

Eclecticism

This refers to the bringing together of knowledge from diverse sources to inform the study and practice of nursing. Eclecticism is concerned with selecting and adapting the best elements from a number of sources to inform curriculum design.

Submissions received by the Forum suggested that a variety of teaching / learning strategies based on theories of teaching and learning should be used in the programme. In deciding on these strategies there is a need to take cognisance of the theories of adult learning as well as the developments in learning technologies, particularly electronic methods of learning. **The Forum recommends that the curriculum design for the nursing degree programme be eclectic insofar as it draws on knowledge from diverse sources and uses a variety of teaching / learning strategies.**

Transferability and Progression

Transferability refers to the need to ensure parity in relation to curricular content and experiences across pre-registration programmes in an attempt to support the notion of transfer between programmes. The principle of transferability also allows students whose primary degree is in general nursing, for instance, to apply for entry to a further registration. Credit would be given for existing courses (modules or units) covered in general nursing and relevant to psychiatric or mental handicap (or vice versa), thereby enhancing a range of clinical pathways. The implementation of the four-year pre-registration degree programme leading to registration as a nurse has implications for the career choices and career paths of nurses. The Commission on Nursing placed particular emphasis on transferability and progression within and between nursing education programmes as well as other third-level courses. However, these issues are complex and require further examination and to this end **the Forum recommends that research be undertaken by An Bord Altranais to examine the issues pertaining to transferability and progression of nursing education programmes leading to registration.**

The application of a modular structure in curriculum design featured in a number of submissions. A module can be described as a self-contained unit of learning with its own aims and learning outcomes and forming part of a programme of study on an educational pathway. The Forum considered the disadvantages as well as advantages of the modular approach. The modular approach has the advantages of flexibility, increased student choice, ease of transfer and progression between programmes and across divisions of the register. It also has certain disadvantages in that it can lead to segmentation and fragmentation of knowledge between modules.

The Forum endorses the principle of transferability and **recommends that a flexible and dynamic approach be adopted to facilitate the transfer and progression of students as far as practicable and suggests that this be considered on an individual basis.**

The Forum welcomes the establishment of a National Qualifications Authority of Ireland under the Qualifications (Education and Training) Act (1999). The objectives of this Act are, *inter alia*, to provide a system for coordinating and comparing education and training awards, to promote procedures for transfer and progression, and to facilitate lifelong learning through the promotion of access and opportunities for all learners. The Forum notes that institutions governed by the Act will be required to inform their students whether the programme of studies they will undertake will be accommodated through the procedures for access, transfer or progression referred to in the Act.

The Forum also notes that in November 1999, the National University of Ireland published a

policy document on an NUI qualifications framework for lifelong learning[23]. The document sets out to establish:-

• an integrated framework of qualifications within the NUI, with transparent paths of progression from the lowest to the highest levels of awards;
• an NUI credit system for certificates and diplomas;
• compatibility of the NUI framework with existing structures of qualifications nationally and with the new national framework to be established under the Authority.

In light of these developments, **the Forum recommends that in the development of curricula for the new four-year degree programme in pre-registration nursing education in Ireland, the National Qualifications Authority and all third-level institutions providing nursing education programmes should ensure that there are transfer pathways in place, thereby enabling nursing students to have the option of changing course specialty, or even to transfer to programmes outside of nursing.**

Utility
Utility refers to the principle that knowledge obtained should be useful in informing the practice of the discipline being studied. The WHO European Strategy for Nursing and Midwifery Education maintains that the content of the curriculum must be relevant to the healthcare priorities and to the epidemiological, demographic and socio-cultural context of the individual member states. The relevance of the sciences and research to the study and practice of nursing is important.

[23] National University of Ireland (1999) *An NUI Qualifications Framework for Lifelong Learning: Access, Progression and Transfer.* Dublin: National University of Ireland.

In submissions to the Forum, the need to integrate nursing theory with nursing practice is reiterated, with the majority highlighting that the exposure of nursing students to clinical learning occurs late into the programme. Earlier clinical experience, more varied supernumerary working patterns and opportunities for learning in community contexts were suggested to enhance learning. Early exposure to practical nursing skills ensures that students can enter placements with credibility and feeling ready for participation. It was also highlighted that a continuous twelve-month clinical placement without any theoretical input would serve to widen the theory-practice gap. To counteract this it is suggested that the primary focus of the rostered placement should be to obtain clinical experience and learn the practice of nursing.

To emphasise clinical as well as theoretical learning and reduce the theory-practice gap **the Forum recommends that clinical placements should be undertaken early in the programme and there should be reflective time built into the rostered year to enhance the consolidation of theory and practice.**

Evidence Base

This principle reflects the view that all aspects of the programme, including its development, delivery and evaluation, need to be grounded in evidence where it exists. The curriculum model needs to promote an open, unbiased search for educationally and clinically sound content, involving all relevant bodies of expertise. Submissions suggest that the degree programme will foster a cadre of critical thinkers in nursing who can access and interpret the findings of relevant evidence therefore **the Forum recommends that the curriculum design for the pre-registration nursing degree programme should have a sound theoretical base.**

Shared Learning

Interdisciplinary and shared learning describe an education that draws from the knowledge and processes of multiple disciplines. As the delivery of healthcare increasingly depends on the effective conjoint working of all healthcare disciplines, it is important that nursing students have the opportunity to interact with other healthcare professionals at an early stage. Shared learning cultivates an ethos of cooperation between disciplines and provides opportunities for enhancing the understanding of each other's roles in healthcare delivery. **The Forum recommends that nursing students should be actively encouraged to learn with and from other healthcare professionals.**

Assessment of Clinical Competence

The measurement of clinical competence is a multidimensional and complex task. In January 1999, An Bord Altranais commenced an exercise in defining competence[24], constructing competencies and validating an assessment strategy. Five broad Domains of Competence and an associated assessment tool are currently being tested in general, psychiatric and mental handicap nursing. A final report on the outcome of this study is expected in December 2000. An Bord Altranais will then use the results of the pilot study to provide further guidance on the assessment of clinical competence.

The resultant Domains of Competence should provide clearer goals for planning the outcomes of the education programme and what is expected of the beginning practitioner. It is important to highlight that the adoption of

---

[24] The Domains of Competence that are currently being piloted are included in Appendix 4 for illustrative purposes. They will be subject to amendment following the results of the pilot study.

Domains of Competence as a requirement to enter An Bord Altranais register does not imply that the Board is advocating a competency-based curriculum. The Forum discussed the concept of a competency-based curriculum and was aware of its limitations in that it is not sufficiently dynamic and holistic and concluded therefore that it is incongruent with the approach and ideals advocated by third-level education.

Curriculum Evaluation and Quality Assurance

Curriculum evaluation is an integral part of curriculum development and is necessary for the success and quality of the entire programme. The WHO European Strategy for Nursing and Midwifery Education recommended that all aspects of the curriculum be planned and evaluated on a regular basis.

At a national level, quality assurance in education is being addressed via the Universities Act (1997), the NCEA Act (1979), the Qualifications (Education and Training) Act (1999) and An Bord Altranais *Requirements and Standards for Nurse Registration Education Programmes* (1999).

The Forum recommends that to ensure a quality education for nursing students all stakeholders, including the students themselves, should be actively involved in the evaluation of the pre-registration nursing degree programme.

Moving from Curriculum Design to Development

Curriculum development is the process of translating curriculum policy statements into an educational programme. The principles which underpin a curriculum should be made explicit and the structures and processes for realising each principle must also be identified. Structures for enabling a principle include material structures (timetables, venues, clinical placements) and non-material structures (communication, decision-making, prioritisation). Processes, which shape attitudes, will determine the conditions for education and will reflect institutional climates or culture. Due to differences in local need, it will always be necessary to establish appropriate structures and processes for implementing principles.

Figure 5.I: Curriculum Overview

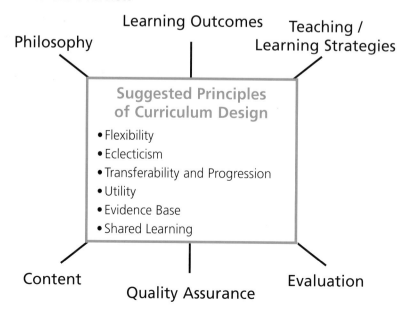

The task for the curriculum development group is to develop a nursing curriculum that has the ability to respond to individual student needs. Figure 5.1 gives an overview of a curriculum with suggested principles of curriculum design at the core of curriculum development. The NEATE Report documented fully the problems that can arise when a partnership approach to curriculum design is not adopted. It is important therefore that all decisions relating to curriculum design, delivery and evaluation are taken jointly by the third-level institutions and the local health service providers and are overseen by the local joint working groups on nursing education.

Recommendations

- The Forum recommends that discussion on the model of professional education to underpin the nursing degree programme should take place between third-level institutions and health service providers.
- The Forum recommends that the curriculum design be dynamic and flexible to permit responsiveness to local needs.
- The Forum recommends that the curriculum design for the nursing degree programme be eclectic insofar as it draws on knowledge from diverse sources and uses a variety of teaching / learning strategies.
- The Forum recommends that research be undertaken by An Bord Altranais to examine the issues pertaining to transferability and progression of nursing education programmes leading to registration.
- The Forum recommends that a flexible and dynamic approach be adopted to facilitate the transfer and progression of students as far as practicable and suggests that this be considered on an individual basis.

- The Forum recommends that in the development of curricula for the new four-year degree programme in pre-registration nursing education in Ireland, the National Qualifications Authority and all third-level institutions providing nursing education programmes should ensure that there are transfer pathways in place, thereby enabling nursing students to have the option of changing course specialty, or even to transfer to programmes outside of nursing.
- The Forum recommends that clinical placements should be undertaken early in the programme and there should be reflective time built into the rostered year to enhance the consolidation of theory and practice.
- The Forum recommends that the curriculum design for the pre-registration nursing degree programme should have a sound theoretical base.
- The Forum recommends that nursing students should be actively encouraged to learn with and from other healthcare professionals.
- The Forum recommends that to ensure a quality education for nursing students all stakeholders, including the students themselves, should be actively involved in the evaluation of the pre-registration nursing degree programme.

The Curriculum -
Learning the Practice of Nursing

Chapter 6

Chapter 6   Key points

- The practice of nursing and clinical learning is an essential part of the nursing curriculum.

- Nursing students need exposure to practice through a range of placements in different settings in which care is delivered.

- Clinical staff have a key role in educating students in the practice of nursing and must be prepared for the role.

- Structures and processes are needed to ensure the integration of theory and practice and effective collaboration between third-level nurse lecturers, students and clinical staff in the practice setting.

Introduction

Learning the practice of nursing is an integral part of the nursing curriculum and the establishment of structures to support student learning in the clinical learning environment is essential. The involvement of all relevant personnel and a partnership approach are the most appropriate and efficient ways to support and maximise clinical learning. Third-level institutions and health service providers must consider and decide on the most appropriate structures and systems to promote high-quality environments for nursing students to learn the practice of nursing.

The clinical learning environment has been defined as *"an interactive network of forces within the clinical setting which influence the nurse's clinical learning outcomes"*[25]. A review of the factors influencing the creation and maintenance of the clinical learning environment[26] was commissioned by the Forum and underpins this chapter.

The main focus of learning within the practice setting is the process of caring for patients and this takes place primarily for students during clinical placements. The identification, selection and auditing of appropriate sites for clinical placements and the allocation of students to these sites are the first tasks to be undertaken. Secondly, the staff must be prepared to support and teach students on clinical placement. Thirdly, the students themselves, whilst on placement, must learn within a structure and process that facilitates their learning and at the same time ensures that quality patient care is maintained.

Organising and Supporting Clinical Placements

Each student must complete a number of general and specialist placements during the degree programme. The task of organising multiple placements, identifying new placements and the associated administrative and practice development work is significant and requires considerable planning and co-ordination between the third-level institution and the health service provider. **The Forum recommends that an allocations function be established in each third-level institution to co-ordinate the placement of students for clinical learning.** The post may or may not be a full-time one, depending on the size of the programme.

This person should liaise with nurse lecturers and health service providers to:-

- ensure that student placement allocations are regularly reviewed and monitored;
- maintain and develop placement areas and identify new placement sites;
- maintain records of placements and student allocations.

Within the health service provider setting, the identification and support of clinical placements will also be an important responsibility. **The Forum recommends that a designated person within each health service provider should be given responsibility to liaise with the responsible person within the third-level institution in relation to clinical placement allocations.** This may not be a full-time post, and will depend on the number of placements to be organised. The person should ideally have a clinical background but the nature and form of this post may vary, depending on local circumstances. The role would involve close liaison with the third-level counterpart and would be mainly concerned with establishing and co-ordinating student placements within the health service

[25] Dunn, S. and Burnett, B. (1995) "The development of a clinical learning environment scale". *Journal of Advanced Nursing*, 22: 1166-1173, page 1166.
[26] McCarthy, M. (2000) *Creating and Maintaining a Clinical Learning Environment*. Dublin: School of Nursing and Midwifery Studies, Trinity College Dublin.

provider. This would be conducted in consultation with the director of nursing and clinical nursing staff and in accordance with An Bord Altranais requirements and standards.

The twelve-month rostered placement, during which the student will be a paid full-time employee of the health services, will have significant implications for the skill mix within the service and requires careful planning. **The Forum recommends that decisions on the allocation of rostered placements should involve particularly close consultation between third-level institutions and health service providers.**

Community Placements

The importance of primary healthcare within health service delivery means that students must have an appropriate level of knowledge and understanding of the community setting. Such knowledge and understanding must be provided in accordance with An Bord Altranais requirements and standards for nurse registration education programmes. Clinical experience should expose the nursing student to the diverse roles and responsibilities of the many and varied personnel involved in care in the community. General nursing students should be facilitated to have further learning opportunities with public health nurses as well as other community experience. Meeting this requirement will require capital investment to develop the necessary facilities for students within the community health centres.

Within the public health nursing structure there are currently no posts analogous to those of nurse practice development co-ordinator or clinical placement co-ordinator. It is clear that some form of educational support and co-ordination is needed to facilitate students'

community placements, the form of which requires further examination. **The Forum recommends a pilot project to explore the need for the clinical placement co-ordinator post within community healthcare.** Such a project could examine, within an urban and a rural community care setting, alternative structural models to facilitate student placements in a community setting. Should the study indicate the need for the appointment of clinical placement co-ordinators or other community staffing structures, this will obviously have cost implications for the health sector.

Clinical Staff Preparation

The need to prepare clinical staff to assume their teaching role in relation to nursing students was emphasised in the NEATE Report and in many of the submissions received. The Forum recognises that this issue is crucial to the integrity of the degree programme and to the successful development of nursing education. The Forum suggests that in-service education would in the short term offer information and guidelines to registered nurses in relation to the pre-registration degree programme.

The Forum recommends that health service providers, in partnership with the relevant third-level institution, should ensure that nurses who support students have attended a teaching and assessing course. It further recommends that within five years of the start of the degree programme all nurses who support students and who have not already completed such a course should have done so.

The Clinical Learning Environment for the Student

Whilst on clinical placement, the nursing student

should receive the requisite support and learning opportunities to facilitate learning the practice of nursing. The student interacts with a range of people, and apart from patients, the roles of the different agents of learning are outlined below:-

The Preceptor

A fundamental component of the role of every nurse is the teaching of nursing students in the practice area. An Bord Altranais recommends that during the clinical placement, the student should be supported by a preceptor, defined as *"a registered nurse who has been specially prepared to guide and direct student learning during clinical placement"*[27]. A preceptor has been defined further as *"an experienced nurse, midwife or health visitor within a practice placement who acts as a role model and resource for a student who is attached to him or her for a specific time span or experience"*[28]. The preceptor also develops a relationship and works closely with the student throughout the placement. **The Forum recommends that each student whilst on clinical placement should be assigned a named preceptor who is a registered nurse.**

The Clinical Nurse Manager

The teaching of pre-registration nursing students is considered to be an integral part of the professional nursing role. The clinical nurse manager has a pivotal role in creating and maintaining a clinical learning environment and can positively influence the attitudes of staff towards the students as well as the quality of the learning experience. It is imperative that this continues to be the case and that the role be further utilised to enhance student learning. **The Forum recommends that the clinical nurse manager continue to have a pivotal role in creating and maintaining a clinical learning environment.**

The Clinical Placement Co-ordinator

Clinical placement co-ordinators were introduced as a mechanism to support students on placement during the introduction of the diploma programme. The Commission on Nursing described them as *"skilled clinical nurses and their role is to guide and support student nurses in assigned clinical areas and to ensure that the clinical placements meet the requirements of the education programme with regard to planned experiences and outcomes"*[29].

A clear distinction can be drawn between the role of a clinical placement co-ordinator and that of a preceptor in relation to student support. The preceptor focuses on the individual student whilst the clinical placement co-ordinator focuses on the placement. The preceptor has a one-to-one relationship with the student and the clinical placement co-ordinator relates to groups of students. The clinical placement co-ordinator has knowledge and experience of a number of placement areas whilst the preceptor has in-depth knowledge of one placement. The preceptor is an integral part of the nursing team involved in the direct delivery of patient care, whilst the clinical placement co-ordinator is supernumerary to the team.

Clinical placement co-ordinators report and are accountable to the nurse practice development co-ordinator. The Commission on Nursing recommended that the role of the clinical placement co-ordinator should be evaluated and this study was in progress as the Forum concluded its deliberations. **The Forum recommends that the role of clinical placement co-ordinator be retained and that the role may be redefined depending on the final results of role evaluation.**

[27] An Bord Altranais (1994) *The Future of Nurse Education and Training in Ireland.* page 26. Dublin: An Bord Altranais.
[28] Quinn, F. (1997) *The Principles and Practice of Nurse Education.* 3rd edition. page 189. Cheltenham: Stanley Thornes (Publishers) Ltd.
[29] Government of Ireland (1998) *Report of the Commission on Nursing: A Blueprint for the Future.* paragraph 5.64. page 91. Dublin: Stationery Office.

The Nurse Practice Development Co-ordinator

The nurse practice development co-ordinator has a wide and varied role that includes responsibility for practice developments and quality assurance in nursing practice. The Commission on Nursing recommended that nurse practice development co-ordinators should oversee the organisation of the pre-registration clinical placements in the health service provider and supervise clinical placement co-ordinators. It is logical therefore that the allocation function outlined above in relation to clinical placements should come under the remit of the nurse practice development co-ordinators.

Third-level Teaching Staff in the Clinical Learning Environment

Teaching staff from third-level institutions, as part of the team in the clinical learning environment, are key in facilitating and contributing to the clinical learning of nursing students. In other countries, and in similar programmes, teaching staff have contributed in a number of ways, including student supervision, tutorials and the provision of advice and direction on aspects of the programme and ensuring liaison and communication between the third-level institution and the clinical site. The presence of teaching staff from the third-level institution in the clinical area is an essential element in implementing the nursing curriculum and in particular ensuring the integration of nursing theory and practice. Many innovative models and arrangements may evolve during the course of curriculum design and programme delivery. An effective arrangement is one where individual lecturers are involved in clinical specialities which are similar to ones where they may have previously practised as clinically based nurses. Matching the clinical specialty of lecturers with their theoretical teaching content makes a very positive contribution to reducing the potential for a theory-practice gap. The use of such a model requires the provision of appropriate time for clinical updating for lecturers and is important to its success. **The Forum recommends that third-level institutions examine opportunities and develop innovative strategies for nurse lecturers to develop their links with clinical areas.**

Joint Appointments in Nursing

Joint appointments between third-level institutions and health service providers, as recommended in the Report of the Commission on Nursing, are considered to be an effective means of reducing the theory-practice gap in nursing education. They also provide a mechanism for strengthening the partnership arrangements between health service providers and the third-level institutions. Joint appointments, whilst of benefit, can be difficult in practice. The Forum considers that joint appointments between third-level institutions and health service providers should be encouraged but suggests that the following guidelines apply in the appointment of staff to these positions:-

- there must be a clear written agreement between both institutions regarding the terms and conditions of the appointment;
- the appointee is selected by both institutions;
- the terms and conditions of the appointment are agreed so that the appointee is clear as to his / her responsibilities;
- the precise type and nature of the written agreement is adapted to meet local needs and circumstances;
- the appointment is reviewed periodically by both institutions with the appointee.

The Forum recommends the development of joint appointments and other innovative strategies to enhance partnership between third-level institutions and health service providers, the precise role and nature of which should be agreed within local partnerships.

Opportunities for Reflection on Practice during the Degree Programme

Clinical learning is enhanced when students are enabled to reflect on their experiences of the clinical practice setting. This is of particular importance during the rostered year. Educational support from lecturers and clinicians is essential to the art of reflection, as is the requirement for protected time out from service delivery. There are many educational strategies that assist the process of reflection on practice including clinical case conferences, paradigm cases, project work, reflective diaries and clinically based tutorials. To emphasise the importance of reflection in learning the practice of nursing, the Forum recommends that within the clinical learning environment all involved should devise innovative and effective ways to maximise the opportunity for students to reflect on and learn from their clinical experience. The Forum recommends that specific periods of protected time be identified for reflection during supernumerary and rostered placements. The amount of time allocated should be agreed formally between third-level institutions and health service providers and included in the memorandum of under-standing.

Recommendations
- The Forum recommends that an allocations function be established in each third-level institution to co-ordinate the placement of students for clinical learning.
- The Forum recommends that a designated person within each health service provider should be given responsibility to liaise with the responsible person within the third-level institution in relation to clinical placement allocations.
- The Forum recommends that decisions on the allocation of rostered placements should involve particularly close consultation between third-level institutions and health service providers.
- The Forum recommends a pilot project to explore the need for the clinical placement co-ordinator post within community health care.
- The Forum recommends that health service providers, in partnership with the relevant third-level institution, should ensure that nurses who support students have attended a teaching and assessing course. It further recommends that within five years of the start of the degree programme all nurses who support students and who have not already completed such a course should have done so.
- The Forum recommends that each student whilst on clinical placement should be assigned a named preceptor who is a registered nurse.
- The Forum recommends that the clinical nurse manager continue to have a pivotal role in creating and maintaining a clinical learning environment.
- The Forum recommends that the role of clinical placement co-ordinator be retained and that the role may be redefined depending on the final results of role evaluation.
- The Forum recommends that third-level

institutions examine opportunities and develop innovative strategies for nurse lecturers to develop their links with clinical areas.

- The Forum recommends the development of joint appointments and other innovative strategies to enhance partnership between third-level institutions and health service providers, the precise role and nature of which should be agreed within local partnerships.

- The Forum recommends that within the clinical learning environment all involved should devise innovative and effective ways to maximise the opportunity for students to reflect on and learn from their clinical experience. The Forum recommends that specific periods of protected time be identified for reflection during supernumerary and rostered placements. The amount of time allocated should be agreed formally between third-level institutions and health service providers and included in the memorandum of understanding.

Costing the Pre-Registration Nursing Degree Programme

Chapter 7

Key points

- Due to data limitations, the Forum can provide only a preliminary estimate of the costs arising from the introduction of the four-year pre-registration nursing degree programme.

- The Forum estimates the average unit cost of the degree programme in 2002 to be £5,300 per student per annum and the total revenue cost to be £57 million in 2002 prices.

- The additional revenue cost of the degree programme, once the diploma costs are offset against it, is estimated at £12.2 million in 2002 prices, an increase of 25% compared to the diploma programme. This figure is subject to revision pending developments in relation to the transfer of nurse teachers and discussions on student meals and the funds available for continuing nurse education.

- A preliminary estimate of the capital investment required is £135 million in 2002 prices but this will require detailed discussions between funding agencies and third-level institutions.

Introduction

One of the Forum's terms of reference was to estimate the additional costs arising from the introduction of a four-year degree programme as a replacement for the three-year diploma programme.

It must be emphasised that the costings outlined in this chapter are a **preliminary estimate**. The true cost of the transition to the degree programme can only be determined following detailed discussions between the stakeholders, a comprehensive review of existing resources within the health and education sectors and analyses of proposals from third-level institutions and associated health service providers for the provision of the degree programme.

Methodology

The Forum decided, in light of limitations in the data available, to cost the proposed degree programme in terms of its additional cost to the Exchequer. Additional in this sense is taken to mean the costs associated with the degree programme less those associated with the diploma programme.

It is important to distinguish between additional costs associated with the transition to a degree programme and those costs associated with a policy decision to increase student numbers. The Department of Health and Children announced its intention to incrementally increase the overall number of nursing students from 3,000 students in 1998 to 4,500 students in 2002 (an intake of 1,500 students for each year of the three-year diploma programme). The proposed increase in the number of nursing students is indicated in Table 7.1.

The Forum adopted a phased approach to identifying the additional revenue cost associated with the introduction of a degree programme. These phases were:-

- identifying expenditure on the existing diploma programme using costing data for the 1997 / 1998 academic year - the only data based on actual financial reports that were available;
- estimating current expenditure on the proposed degree programme;
- projecting this expenditure forward to 2002 using agreed inflators;

Table 7.1:   **Number of Nursing Students during Transition from the Diploma Programme to the Degree Programme**

Year	Student Complement on the Diploma Programme	Student Complement on the Degree Programme
2000	3,500	-
2001	4,000	-
2002	3,000	1,500
2003	1,500	3,000
2004	A small number who have not completed the diploma programme	4,500
2005	-	6,000

- adjusting the expenditure estimates to take account of the fact that the student intake per year in 1998 was approximately 1,000 while the proposed student intake in 2002 will be 1,500 per annum.

The 2002 costs were projected from the 1997 / 1998 base costs using agreed rates for the student maintenance and book grants for 2000, October 2000 salary costs in the health sector, a preliminary estimate of 1999 / 2000 unit costs in the Higher Education Authority (HEA) sector based on 21% pay inflation and 9% non-pay inflation since 1997 / 1998 and by applying inflators which are currently used by the Department of Finance to agree funding across Departments. These inflators are as follows:

Pay   2001: 5.5%   Non-Pay   2001: 3.5%
      2002: 4.0%   2002: 2.3%

The potential capital costs associated with the introduction of a degree programme were dealt with separately. There may be a requirement for initial start-up funding in respect of the degree programme, for example, in the development of library supports. These are capital costs, however, and it is not possible to estimate these costs in the absence of detailed proposals from third-level institutions and a detailed analysis of the existing level of academic supports for students in third-level institutions.

It should be noted that these cost estimates do not include any provision for the cost of the implementation structures alluded to in Chapter 4, namely the national implementation committee, the inter-departmental steering committee, the local joint working groups or the project managers and their associated support staff.

Details of all calculations to generate projected 2002 estimates are included in Appendix 5.

Information Sources

In order to estimate the level of current expenditure on the diploma programme the Forum commissioned a research study[30]. Its terms of reference were to:-

- determine the cost of the Registration / Diploma in Nursing;
- estimate the total resources available, in a single calendar year, to nursing education, in respect of the Registration / Diploma in Nursing for the provision of the three years of the programme;
- prepare and present a report of the findings to the Forum.

The report was submitted to the Forum in December 1999 and presented estimates of the costs of the diploma programme in the 1997 / 1998 academic year. In the absence of full costing data from the Department of Health and Children in respect of the diploma programme, the Forum had to base its estimates on the data generated by the research. It was, however, aware that there is no standard process across health boards and schools of nursing in the way cost centres are dealt with. Accounting and budgetary systems differed and data were not always easy to collect or compare. For that reason the estimates must be regarded as preliminary.

Funding Structures

Recommendations of the Commission on Nursing

The Commission on Nursing recommended that funding for the degree in nursing should remain

---

[30] Carney, M. (1999) "An Analysis of the Costing of the Registration / Diploma in Nursing in the Republic of Ireland". Dublin: School of Nursing and Midwifery, University College Dublin.

initially with the Department of Health and Children and should become the responsibility of the Minister for Education and Science once nursing education is integrated into the third-level sector.

The Commission also called for the funding for the degree programme given to the Department of Education and Science to be red circled until the degree programme is well established. This red circling of funding has been endorsed by the third-level institutions. The Forum endorses the Commission's recommendations regarding the red circling of funding for the pre-registration nursing degree programme.

Funding Structures during the Transition Phase

The policy decisions concerning the overall funding of the degree programme will continue to be made during the transition phase by the Minister for Health and Children, in consultation with the Ministers for Education and Science and Finance. It may not be considered practical for the Department of Health and Children to replicate for such a short time-frame all aspects of the existing funding and payment structures within the education sector. The Forum has therefore recommended the establishment of an inter-departmental steering committee as referred to in Chapter 4 to consider all funding issues associated with the introduction of the degree programme.

Funding for the health service providers in respect of expenses incurred as a result of taking students on supernumerary clinical placements and for the rostered clinical year, such as the provision of uniforms, should remain within the general funding for health service providers. As student numbers increase, such funding will need to increase accordingly. This expenditure will not become the responsibility of the Minister for Education and Science as it relates to the operational expenses incurred by health service providers and not to the expenses incurred by the third-level institutions.

Estimated Revenue Cost of the Diploma Programme

The research commissioned by the Forum examined the current level of funding associated with the pre-registration diploma in nursing by sending questionnaires to each participating school of nursing and third-level institution. These were followed up by a number of meetings and telephone contacts with third-level institutions and schools of nursing.

The research report estimated the recurrent cost of the diploma programme to be £33.8m in the 1997 / 1998 academic year for 2,967 students. It comprised the elements indicated in Table 7.2 overleaf.

Estimated Revenue Cost of the Proposed Degree Programme

The estimated revenue cost of the proposed degree programme can be divided into four components:-

- cost of the rostered clinical year;
- unit cost of the three academic years to the education sector;
- maintenance grant paid to nursing students;
- cost of clinical placement co-ordinators.

Cost of the Rostered Clinical Year

There are three components to the cost of the rostered clinical year, namely, (a) the salaries paid to students, (b) the professional support for students during clinical placements and (c) the unit cost to the education sector of the rostered clinical year.

(a) Salaries Paid to Students

The Commission on Nursing recommended that students undertake a period of twelve months continuous clinical placement as paid employees of the health service and be paid at the rate of 80% of the first-year salary of a staff nurse. It is anticipated that the costing profile of the twelve-month rostered clinical placement will also cover the clinical support costs (primarily clinical placement co-ordinators) associated with super-numerary clinical placements.

The Forum decided at the outset to separate the twelve-month rostered clinical placement from the rest of the degree programme for costing purposes as there were no readily comparable courses in the third-level sector. Also the rostered placement raises issues in relation to costs which do not arise in relation to the academic element of the programme and the use of salaried nursing students as part of the nursing workforce has service implications.

The Forum, in calculating the estimated additional cost of paying students during their rostered clinical placement, decided to use the existing formula in place for the final fourteen weeks of clinical placement in the pre-registration diploma programme. This formula has been in operation for a number of years and provides for a student-staff nurse replacement ratio of 2:1. The formula was adjusted slightly to reflect annual leave, sick leave and reflective time during the twelve-month rostered clinical placement[32]. The additional cost of paying a salary to 1,500 nursing students for twelve-month rostered clinical placements, based on this formula is estimated at £16.9m in 2002 projected prices.

Table 7.2:   Estimated Revenue Cost of the Diploma Programme, 1997 / 1998

Salaries of nurse teachers and others	£7.0m
Salaries of clinical placement co-ordinators	£2.8m
Marginal cost to nursing schools of running the diploma programme	£2.0m
Library costs	£0.9m
Maintenance grants to students	£9.7m
Free meals to students	£3.6m
Book grants for students	£0.2m
Fees paid to third-level institutions	£3.6m
Third-level costs not covered by fees	£0.5m
Salaries of students on rostered clinical placement	£2.3m
Miscellaneous[31]	£1.2m
Total Estimated Expenditure in 1997 / 1998	**£33.8m**

[31] The miscellaneous costs include such items as travel expenses, laundry and photocopying.

[32] Formula to calculate additional salary costs in the rostered clinical year for students: [n/2 x (80% of first-year nurse salary)] + 22% for premium payments + 12.5% PRSI + 20% in respect of cover for annual and sick leave and reflective time.

The environment into which nursing students may be placed has altered radically in recent years. Nursing shortages and increased specialisation in the health services require that the student-staff nurse replacement ratio be examined in detail against the background of anticipated changes in the health services. Nursing students will not be placed on twelve-month rostered placement until 2005 at the earliest. This provides the Department of Health and Children with an opportunity to carry out further research into the student-staff replacement ratio of 2:1. **The Forum recommends that the Department of Health and Children engage external consultants at the earliest opportunity to examine in detail all aspects of the student-staff ratio during the twelve-month rostered clinical placement.**

(b) Professional Support for Students during Clinical Placements

Students will require support and guidance whilst on clinical placement. Much of this support is already in place. The "preceptoring" of students is already an inherent part of the role of every nurse in the clinical environment, hence no additional salary costs will arise from the "preceptoring", support and guidance given to students during their clinical placements. In addition, clinical placement co-ordinators are in place to support the clinical placement of students during the pre-registration diploma programme.

Whilst it is recognised that the "preceptoring" of students is an inherent part of the role of all nurses, it is also recognised that such a role would be enhanced through the preparation of staff in teaching and assessing as indicated in Chapter 6. This programme of preparation will give rise to staff replacement costs. It is not possible to estimate at this stage the likely cost of such a preparation programme. Of the 27,000 nurses in the public health sector, it is not known how many will have already completed a teaching and assessing course prior to the roll-out of a dedicated programme. The duration of various teaching and assessing courses might vary and the extent to which nursing education centres and nurse teachers who choose to remain in the health sector would deliver such courses is not yet clear. If a programme of preparation were rolled out over a period of five years, the costs associated with such a programme would need to take account of replacement costs and lecturer rates.

The sum of £8.5 million was made available by the Department of Health and Children in 1999 to health service providers for the continuing education of nurses. Additional funding was also allocated to the Department of Health and Children in 2000 for continuing nursing education. Clearly there will be a cost attached to any training provided to staff nurses and clinical nurse managers to assist in supporting degree students in the clinical environment. This cost will include both the replacement costs and the fees to be paid to the providers of such training support.

The Forum recommends that priority be accorded by health service providers to the provision of preceptorship training for clinical nursing staff. If the existing resources are inadequate for this purpose, then a case should be made by individual providers to the Department of Health and Children for additional funding for this particular form of training, based on an analysis of existing expenditure on continuing nursing education.

(c) Unit Cost to the Education Sector of the Rostered Clinical Year

The question of an amount to be paid to third-level institutions whilst students are on twelve-month rostered clinical placement was considered by the Forum. The rationale for the rostered clinical year is the acquisition of clinical skills and the further integration of theory and practice to ensure that students can register with An Bord Altranais as competent practitioners on completion of the degree programme. The Forum recognises that there will be a cost to the third-level institutions in respect of nursing students' access to general facilities and in the, albeit reduced, contact time with third-level staff during the clinical year. Therefore, the Forum has used a unit costing for the third-level institutions of £1,900 per student per annum as an estimate for costing the clinical year in 2002. This roughly equates to the annual amount currently paid to the third-level institutions for the services they provide as part of the diploma programme (i.e. £1,500 per student per annum), projected forward to 2002 prices.

The unit costing for this element of the educational programme as delivered by the third-level institutions is added to the unit costing estimated for the other three years of the degree programme (as outlined below) to provide an average for the four years. Unit costings averaged across the four years of the programme will be used as the basis for discussions on the funding for the programme with the third-level institutions. The funding for this element of the clinical rostered year will become the responsibility of the Minister for Education and Science.

Unit Cost of the Three Academic Years to the Education Sector

The Forum also examined unit costs per student at undergraduate level, which are collected annually by the HEA in respect of the university colleges. The HEA's unit costings encompass salary costs (which comprise approximately 75% of the total unit costings) and all other recurrent costs such as those associated with library, information technology, catering and recreational facilities. The student tuition fees, which the third-level institutions receive as income, are accounted for in these unit costs.

The Department of Education and Science does not currently use a unit cost system for assessing the funding requirements of the Institutes of Technology. While there were no unit cost data available in relation to the Institutes of Technology, the Forum felt that the data available from the HEA would nonetheless allow it to produce an indicative costing of the overall programme as delivered by both sectors.

Average unit costs for undergraduate academic groupings (roughly equivalent to faculties) as collated by the HEA in respect of the university colleges in 1997 / 1998 were as follows:-

Arts	£3,700
Business	£3,400
Science	£5,100
Engineering	£5,500
Medicine	£5,000

In looking at unit costs it was considered more appropriate to look at averages for the various academic groupings, as a preliminary analysis of course costs indicated considerable variations between universities at individual course level, which are due to a number of local and other factors. The following examples are cited for illustrative purposes.[33]

[33] Source: Higher Education Authority.

	University (A)	University (B)
	£	£
Bachelor of Medicine	4,400	5,000
Bachelor of Physiotherapy	4,800	6,500
Bachelor of Radiography	8,000	4,100

Whilst no specific comparator is recommended, the Forum concluded that, given the laboratory and practical elements of the nursing degree course and the scale of student numbers involved, an annual unit cost of £5,000 per student would be appropriate based on figures above for the 1997 / 1998 academic year. This was projected forward to approximately £6,400, per student, per annum, at 2002 prices.

It is emphasised that this figure should only be used for estimating the cost associated with the introduction of the pre-registration nursing degree programme. The actual individual unit costs will be subject to local negotiations and are likely to vary somewhat across both the HEA and Institute of Technology sectors due to local circumstances.

State funding of third-level courses is provided without reference to staff-student ratios. It will be a matter for the third-level institutions to design programmes to satisfy the requirements of An Bord Altranais and to ensure the accreditation by An Bord Altranais of course graduates.

In calculating the overall recurrent cost, the unit cost for the three academic years of the programme in 2002 is estimated at £6,400, while a unit costing of £1,900 has been associated with the marginal cost associated with students' access to general college facilities and the reduced level of contact with academic staff during the twelve-month rostered clinical placement. This gives an average unit cost to be

applied for the four years of the programme of £5,300 per student, per annum, in 2002 prices.

This unit cost multiplied by 6,000 students gives a preliminary estimated revenue cost for a pre-registration nursing degree programme of £31.8m on the basis of unit costs for 1997 / 1998 projected forward into 2002.

Maintenance Grant Paid to Nursing Students
The Commission on Nursing recommended that any student benefits available to nursing students should be the same as those available to other third-level students. This recommendation has implications for the current level of grant support offered to nursing students. This grant support is far more generous than that available to the general body of students. Nursing students currently receive an annual non-means tested maintenance grant of £3,325. Nursing students also receive a range of additional supports such as free meals and book grants that are not available to other third-level students.

The maintenance grant available to general third-level students is means tested on the basis of the student's parents' income. There are two levels of grant currently available depending on the distance of the student's parents' home from the third-level institution. The adjacent rate is currently (2000 / 2001) £705 per annum and the non-adjacent rate is £1,765 per annum. Approximately 40% of third-level students qualify for maintenance grants. Of those who presently receive the grant, 25% do so at the adjacent rate and 75% at the non-adjacent rate. Those eligible for the maintenance grant are also eligible for alleviation of the student services charge. This was set at £290 for the 2000 / 2001 academic year. Clearly, no maintenance grant will be payable to salaried students on their twelve-month rostered clinical placement.

On the assumption that nursing students will follow this pattern, it is estimated that the additional cost of encompassing 4,500 nursing students within the maintenance grant scheme, would amount to £3.4m at projected 2002 rates.

Funding will be given to the health agencies, as part of their overall block grant, for providing uniforms to supernumerary students and giving assistance, where appropriate, with travel costs. These operational expenses will occur as a result of taking students on supernumerary clinical placements. The health agencies must consider the standard of service to patients and discharge their responsibilities under health and safety legislation. Such assistance is already provided by health agencies to nursing students. It should be noted that these expenses which relate to supernumerary clinical placements would not be incurred during the twelve-month rostered clinical placement for which the student is salaried and as such will not require funding for that period.

Cost of Clinical Placement Co-ordinators

The unit costings for the third-level academic programme identified in the preceding section exclude the salary costs of clinical placement co-ordinators, who will remain employees of the health services. Research commissioned by the Forum identified 116 clinical placement co-ordinators in 1997 / 1998. The Department of Health and Children estimates that this number will increase to 150 in 2002 at a projected cost of £4.9m. This figure does not include the possible creation of new clinical placement co-ordinator posts in the community care setting. The Forum has recommended that a pilot project be undertaken to explore the utility of the clinical placement co-ordinator post in the community.

Conclusion: Estimated Revenue Cost of Proposed Degree Programme

The estimated revenue costs of a four-year pre-registration nursing degree programme are indicated in Table 7.3.

The estimated total cost of a four-year pre-registration degree programme on the basis of the previously identified assumptions is thus £57m, at 2002 prices, taking account of the proposed increase in the number of students.

The Additional Cost of Introducing the Degree Programme

The additional cost of introducing the degree programme is the difference between the cost of the diploma programme and the cost of the degree programme. However, some of the costs associated with the diploma programme are not readily transferable to the degree programme. In order to identify the additional cost of the degree programme it is necessary to identify those items of expenditure in the diploma programme that will not recur in the degree programme and can be offset against the cost of the degree programme.

The costs associated with the diploma programme that may be offset against the costs of the degree programme are:-

* salaries of clinical placement co-ordinators who are currently involved in the provision of the diploma programme and who will also be involved in the degree programme;
* the salaries of nurse teachers who choose to transfer to the third-level sector;
* payments to the third-level sector for the existing diploma programme;

- the non-means tested support grant of £3,325 per student which will be withdrawn and substituted by a means-tested maintenance grant;
- student book grants which will be withdrawn;
- student meals which will no longer be provided by health service providers;
- student salaries whilst on fourteen-week rostered placement plus other miscellaneous costs[34].

The directors of finance of the health boards queried the figure spent on meals for nursing students. It was suggested this figure did not reflect the marginal cost of the provision of meals for students. In the absence of alternative costings or other empirical data the Forum had to proceed on the basis of the information supplied in the research report. However, **the Forum recommends that discussions should take place between the Departments of Finance and Health and Children and health service providers on the extent, if any, to which funding on student meals may be offset against the additional cost of the degree programme.**

It must be emphasised that this is a preliminary estimate of offset costs and is subject to further discussions and decisions on certain key variables. These include:-

- the number of nurse teachers who transfer from the health sector to the third-level education sector;
- further clarification on the costs associated with student meals;
- clarification on issues relating to current expenditure on continuing nurse education.

Combining the projected offset costs for the diploma in 2002 with the figures in Table 7.3, the additional revenue cost of the degree programme in 2002 prices is estimated in Table 7.4 overleaf.

These estimates are in 2002 prices. The purpose of the estimate is to show how much more the degree programme will cost, compared to the diploma programme. This does not mean that they are an estimate of the projected actual cost of the degree programme in 2002. They are rather an indicative cost estimate of what the degree programme might cost were it to be fully

Table 7.3   Estimated Revenue Cost of the Degree Programme at 2002 Prices

Estimated Revenue Costs (2002 Prices)	
Cost of third-level academic programme (unit cost to third-level sector of 6,000 students)	£31.8m
Additional cost of twelve-month rostered clinical placement (student salaries)	£16.9m
Student maintenance grant	£3.4m
Salaries of clinical placement co-ordinators	£4.9m
Total Estimated Cost of Pre-registration Degree Programme (2002 prices)	**£57.0m**

[34] Only 50% of these additional miscellaneous costs are offset.

operational in 2002 with the full complement of 6,000 students, 1,500 of them on rostered placement. The reality is of course, as Table 7.1 indicates, that it is not until 2005 that the degree programme will reach its full complement of 6,000 students. In 2002 there will be only 1,500 degree students and 3,000 students completing the diploma programme. Table 7.4 thus compares the preliminary estimate, in 2002 prices, of the diploma programme as compared to the degree programme.

The estimated additional revenue cost of introducing a degree in projected 2002 comparative costing terms, is £12.2m. Therefore, the introduction of a degree programme in 2002 will, in revenue costing terms, on the basis of the information available to the Forum, cost approximately 25% more than the diploma programme. This is based on student numbers of 6,000, with 1,500 on rostered clinical placement for twelve months.

Estimated Capital Cost of the Proposed Nursing Degree Programme

The capital cost of the proposed degree programme has two components, pensions and physical capital.

Pensions[36]

Four of the universities operate funded pension schemes while Institutes of Technology operate under the Local Government Superannuation Act (1980).

Table 7.4:   Estimated Additional Revenue Cost of the Degree Programme at 2002 Prices

Diploma Offset Costs (for 4,500 students: 1,500 over 3 years)		Degree Costs (for 6,000 students: 1,500 over 4 years)	
Salaries of nurse tutors (estimated number of nurse tutors in 2002 = 225)	£8.2m	Cost of third-level academic programme (unit cost to third-level sector of 6,000 students)	£31.8m
Third-level fees and costs	£5.5m	Additional cost of twelve-month rostered clinical placement (student salaries)	£16.9m
Student maintenance grant	£15.8m	Student maintenance grant	£3.4m
Salaries of clinical placement co-ordinators	£4.9m	Salaries of clinical placement co-ordinators	£4.9m
Student book grants	£0.5m		
Student meals[35]	£6.2m		
Student salaries	£3.0m		
Miscellaneous	£0.7m		
Total	**£44.8m**	**Total**	**£57.0m**

[35] Subject to further discussions as recommended in this report.
[36] Pensions are treated as a capital cost in this estimate because they are a non-recurrent cost.

There would be no pension cost associated with nurse teachers transferring to Institutes of Technology. The scheme, as operated by the Department of the Environment and Local Government (it is planned to transfer the operation soon to the Department of Education and Science), would involve the transfer of pension entitlements and not require any capital investment. Similarly, there is no capital cost associated with the transfer of staff to two of the universities.

There would be a pension cost associated with nurse teachers transferring as employees to four of the universities. The research report commissioned by the Forum identified 240 nurse teachers involved in the pre-registration diploma programme in 1998. It is difficult to estimate at this stage the numbers of nurse teachers who are likely to transfer to the third-level sector. There is, as yet, no formal indication of the numbers of nurse teachers who will transfer to the third-level sector. However, for the purposes of the preliminary estimated costings it is assumed that 160 nurse teachers will transfer and that of those 100 will transfer to third-level institutions with funded schemes. The exact amount that would need to be paid into a scheme to preserve a person's pension entitlements depends on their age and length of service. The Forum obtained an estimate of £75,000 per person transferring into a funded scheme based on an agreed profile of the age and service of transferees. These assumptions produce a cost estimate of £7.5m. This figure will need to be adjusted should the actual number of nurse teachers who transfer be greater or lesser than the estimate above. The actual amount to be paid into a scheme would be a matter for the trustees of the pension funds concerned and would be paid at the time of transfer.

Physical Capital

The Commission on Nursing *"considered that nursing students should be educated to degree level and be fully integrated within the third-level education sector"*[37]. It also indicated that it was *"conscious that the integration of nursing students onto the campuses of third-level institutes may require substantial capital investment"*[38]. Costings for the capital cost of a degree programme are estimated on the basis of a projected pre-registration nursing student population of 6,000. 1,500 of these students would be on twelve-month rostered clinical placement in the health sector and as such, will not require "full integration" within the third-level sector.

The Forum explored the issue of capital costings on the assumption that all 4,500 nursing students would need to be accommodated (in terms of lecture theatres, library and IT facilities, and so on) for the full duration of the programme in new buildings on the main campuses of the third-level institutions.

The Forum estimated that such a scenario would involve a capital investment requirement of approximately £135m. This estimate is for 2002 prices and is based on discussions members of the Forum had with officials from the Planning and Building Unit of the Department of Education and Science. This does not include any allowance for the maintenance of buildings. The main assumption underlying this estimate is that the full integration of nursing students within the third-level sector would require the provision of lecture facilities for nursing students for the entire duration of their course (excluding the clinical year) on the main educational campus. This capital requirement could be reduced by the fact that some accommodation is

[37] Government of Ireland (1998) *Report of the Commission on Nursing: A Blueprint for the Future*. paragraph 5.19. page 7. Dublin: Stationery Office.
[38] *Ibid.*, paragraph 5.42. page 8.

already provided on some of the main third-level campuses for nursing diploma students. It could also be reduced somewhat by the time-tabling of clinical placements. It would be incumbent on each third-level institution to demonstrate the extent to which academic integration would require the physical integration of capital facilities within the main campus.

In addition, the increased use of community clinical placements as discussed in Chapter 6 may have capital cost implications. These costs are not included in the estimates and should be the subject of further discussion.

The planning of the capital investment programme should be a matter for the inter-departmental steering committee, taking policy direction from the Ministers for Health and Children, Education and Science and Finance, with input from the national implementation committee. The provision of such a substantial capital investment programme will require careful planning and phasing over the medium to long term.

Recommendations

- The Forum recommends that the Department of Health and Children engage external consultants at the earliest opportunity to examine in detail all aspects of the student-staff ratio during the twelve-month rostered clinical placement.
- The Forum recommends that priority be accorded by health service providers to the provision of preceptorship training for clinical nursing staff. If the existing resources are inadequate for this purpose, then a case should be made by individual providers to the Department of Health and Children for additional funding for this particular form of training, based on an analysis of existing expenditure on continuing nursing education.
- The Forum recommends that discussions should take place between the Departments of Finance and Health and Children and health service providers on the extent, if any, to which funding on student meals may be offset against the additional cost of the degree programme.

To Conclude…

To Conclude...

The dawn of this new century brings with it significant challenges for nursing and nursing education. Nursing now has a tremendous opportunity to shape its own future. It is about changing and moving on from the past and moving to the opportunities that now present so that the nursing profession can grow.

Ireland is currently experiencing a historical low unemployment rate. While nursing has long been an occupational group subject to swings in supply and demand, the current gap between the need for nurses and their supply, is forcing health service providers to look at new initiatives and innovative ways of attracting and retaining nursing personnel within the Irish health services. This is the most immediate challenge for the profession.

The sustained focus on partnership and co-operation between the various stakeholders represented on the Forum during the course of its deliberations has led to a greater level of understanding and appreciation of each other's role and function in the provision of nursing education. This positive, co-operative spirit augurs well for the implementation of the pre-registration nursing degree programme and for the profession of nursing.

Undergraduate nursing education will always need development and redesign to meet the requirements of the system. The future is partnership and nursing must be capable of responding to changing health needs, interdisciplinary practice and education, technological advances, expanding multiculturalism and the globalisation of healthcare. The recommendations in this report are designed to provide an enabling educational infrastructure, founded on the principle of partnership, one within which the profession can evolve. The process of partnership has already commenced. It is critical that this continues to ensure that nursing and nursing education can flourish and respond adequately to the range of issues facing the Irish health sector.

The ultimate success of the changes in nursing education must be judged, however, in terms of the quality of care experienced by those who require nursing care.

Appendices

Appendix 1

Submissions Received

1. Mental Health and Social Care Research Group.
2. School of Nursing, St James's Hospital, Dublin.
3. Martha McGinn, Clinical Placement Co-ordinator, St Joseph's Hospital, Clonsilla, Dublin.
4. COPE Foundation Nurses.
5. Health Sciences Libraries Group of the Library Association of Ireland.
6. Clinical Placement Co-ordinators, St James's Hospital, Dublin.
7. Nurse Teachers, c/o School of Nursing and Midwifery, Trinity Centre for Health Sciences, St James's Hospital, Dublin.
8. College of Nursing, Adelaide & Meath Hospital, Dublin, Incorporating The National Children's Hospital.
9. Clinical Placement Co-ordinators, James Connolly Memorial Hospital, Blanchardstown.
10. Irish Nursing Research Interest Group.
11. National Council for Vocational Awards.
12. Centre for Nursing Studies, National University of Ireland, Galway.
13. European Cranial & Complementary Medical Association (for Practitioners working within Prisons).
14. Irish Nurses Organisation.
15. Gaellinn.
16. Irish Nursing Practice Development Co-ordinators Association.
17. School of Nursing, St Ita's Hospital, Portrane, Co. Dublin.
18. Nursing Staff, University College Hospital, Galway.
19. National Rehabilitation Hospital, Dun Laoghaire.
20. National Superintendent Public Health Nurses Group.
21. Nurse Tutors, Cork University Hospital.
22. Nursing Staff, Cork University Hospital.
23. Patrick Murray, Letterkenny General Hospital, Letterkenny, Co. Donegal.
24. John Birthistle, St Michael's House, Ballymun, Dublin.
25. School of Nursing, St Vincent's Hospital, Elm Park, Dublin.
26. Clinical Placement Co-ordinators, Beaumont Hospital, Dublin.
27. Clinical Placement Co-ordinators, Mercy, South Infirmary, Victoria Hospitals, Cork.
28. An Bord Altranais.
29. Medical Library, University College Dublin.
30. School of Psychiatric Nursing, Southern Health Board.
31. Department of Nursing, University College Cork.
32. Multi-disciplinary Group, St James's Hospital, Dublin.
33. David Kieran, Sisters of the Sacred Hearts of Jesus and Mary, St Anne's, Roscrea, Co. Tipperary.
34. Social and Community Care Department, Cork College of Commerce.
35. Nora O'Callaghan, Mater Misericordiae Hospital, Dublin.
36. Staff Nurses, Midland Regional School of Nursing, Tullamore, Co. Offaly.
37. Anne Buckley, Outpatients' Department, Beaumont Hospital, Dublin.
38. Ward Sister, St Pius' Ward, University College Hospital, Galway.
39. Ward Sister and Staff Nurses, St Nicholas' Ward, University College Hospital, Galway.

40. Tutors of Cork Voluntary Hospitals, School of Nursing, c/o Mercy Hospital, Cork.

41. Clinical Placement Co-ordinators, Waterford Regional Hospital.

42. Mary McHugh, Margaret Cooke, Lisa Walsh, Portiuncula Hospital, Ballinasloe, Co. Galway.

43. Richard Deady, Southern Health Board, Our Lady's Hospital, Cork.

44. Tutorial Staff , School of Nursing, Sligo General Hospital, Sligo.

45. Nurse Tutors, Beaumont Hospital, Dublin.

46. Violet Hayes, West Cork Community Care, Skibbereen, Co. Cork.

47. Nurse Tutors, Mater Misericordiae Hospital, Dublin.

48. Liz Dunbar, The Children's Hospital, Temple Street, Dublin.

49. Care Alliance Ireland.

50. School of Nursing, Our Lady's Hospital for Sick Children, Crumlin, Dublin.

51. Hospitaller Order of St John of God, Stillorgan, Co. Dublin.

52. Nurse Tutors & Clinical Teachers Section, Irish Nurses Organisation.

53. Emer Ward, The Children's Hospital, Temple Street, Dublin.

54. St Louise's School of Nursing, St. Joseph's Hospital, Clonsilla, Dublin.

55. Nurses of COPE Foundation, Occupational Centre, Glasheen, Cork.

56. Mark Philbin, St Vincent's Psychiatric Hospital, Fairview, Dublin.

57. Nursing Executive Group, Mater Misericordiae Hospital, Dublin.

58. St Vincent's Hospital and Area 7 Psychiatric Services, Fairview, Dublin.

59. Jim Callaghan, St Angela's College of Education, Sligo.

60. Faculty of Nursing and Midwifery, Royal College of Surgeons in Ireland, Dublin.

61. School of Nursing, Regional Hospital, Limerick.

62. Nurse Tutors, College of Nursing, Mater Misericordiae Hospital, Dublin. (second submission)

63. School of Nursing and Midwifery, University College Dublin.

64. School of Nursing, Dublin City University.

Appendix 2

Expert Advisers and Consultations

1. Dr Martin Newell, Director, Central Applications Office, Galway.

2. Ms Niamh O'Donoghue, Principal Officer, Local Appointments Commission.

3. Professor Helen Simons, University of Southampton.

4. Professor Áine Hyland, Chairperson and Mr Seán Ó Foghlú, Secretary, The Points Commission.

5. An Bord Altranais Education Committee.

6. Professor Oliver Slevin, CEO, National Board for Nursing, Midwifery and Health Visiting, Northern Ireland.

7. Nurse Tutors, Nursing Management, Nursing Practice Development Co-ordinator, Clinical Placement Co-ordinators, Traditional and Diploma Students, Our Lady of Lourdes Hospital, Drogheda.

8. Nurse Tutors, Nursing Management, Clinical Placement Co-ordinators, Traditional and Diploma Students, Clinical Staff, St Mary's Hospital, Drumcar, Co. Louth.

9. Nursing Executive, Nurse Tutors, Clinical Placement Co-ordinators, Diploma Students, Mater Misericordiae Hospital, Dublin.

10. Teaching Staff, Nurse Tutors, Nursing Management, Nursing Practice Development Co-ordinator, Clinical Placement Co-ordinators, General and Psychiatry Diploma Students, Waterford Institute of Technology.

11. Mental Health and Social Care Research Group.

12. Professor Jean Orr, Director, The School of Nursing and Midwifery, The Queen's University of Belfast, Belfast.

13. Ms Judith Hill, Chief Nursing Officer, Department of Health and Social Services, Northern Ireland.

14. Professor Jenny Boore, Co-ordinator of Academic Affairs, The University of Ulster, Belfast.

15. Professor Betty Kershaw, Dean, School of Nursing, Midwifery and Health Visiting, University of Sheffield.

16. Ms Roisin Kellegher, President, Institute of Guidance Counsellors.

17. Clinical Placement Co-ordinators Association.

18. Irish Nursing Practice Development Co-ordinators Association.

19. Nursing Alliance.

20. Mr David Coghlan, University of Dublin, School of Business Studies, Trinity College, Dublin.

21. Registrars and Bursars of Universities / Colleges.

22. Directors of Institutes of Technology.

23. Nursing Teaching Staff in third-level institutions involved in pre-registration nursing education.

24. Mr Martin McDonald, Health Services Employers Agency.

25. Professor Patricia Benner, Department of Psychological Nursing, University of California, San Francisco.

26. The Paediatric Nurse Education Review Group.

27. Mr Jonathan Drennan, Lecturer, Faculty of Nursing and Midwifery, Royal College of Surgeons in Ireland.

Appendix 3

Sample Memorandum of Understanding between (health service provider) and (third-level institution)

1. General Context:
In the context of the Nurses' Act (1985), the Universities Act (1997), the NCEA Act (1979), the Regional Technical Colleges' Act (1992 and 1999), the Qualifications Act (1999) and the regulations associated with this legislation, and taking account of the Nurses' Rules, 1988 (Amendment) Rules, 1998 and 1999, this Memorandum of Understanding is hereby agreed by (health service provider) and (third-level institution) in relation to the operation of the four-year pre-registration Degree programme in (General/Psychiatric/Mental Handicap) Nurse Education. This Memorandum applies to all such education programmes commencing in or after September 2002.

2. Legislative Framework:
2.1 (Health service provider) and (third-level institution) recognise the legislative requirements in relation to nursing education and registration, assessments and examinations specified in the Nurses Act (1985) and undertake to operate in accordance with that legislation and any Rules made by An Bord Altranais thereunder or any future legislation and Rules in respect of nursing education, examinations and registration.

2.2 (Health service provider) recognises the statutory obligations of (third-level institution/awarding authority) in respect of its approval of programmes for (third level institution) awards, as specified in the (relevant legislation governing the third-level institution).

3. Partnership Arrangements:
The Degree programme is being conducted in partnership between (health service provider) and (third-level institution/awarding authority). Responsibility for the education of students, both theoretical and clinical, lies with (third-level institution). Responsibility for the provision and supervision of clinical experience lies with (health service provider). Academic staff from (third-level institution) will be covered for liability in accordance with the insurance policy of (health service provider) while engaged in clinical teaching or assessing of students or while updating their own clinical skills in the premises of (health service provider).

4. Co-operative Structures:
A (Department/School/Centre/Faculty) of (Nursing/Nursing Studies/Nursing and Midwifery) has been established in (third-level institution) to manage the programme, to co-ordinate the theoretical content with the statutory clinical content, including the rostered year, and to provide the necessary administrative support system. A Director, who holds a nursing qualification, has been appointed as head of the (Department/School/Centre/Faculty) of (Nursing/Nursing Studies/Nursing and Midwifery)

5. Joint Working Group:
A relevant joint working group (has been/will be) established, with balanced representation from (third-level institution) and (health service provider), to monitor the progress of the programme. Chairperson(s) will be agreed by the working group. Sub committees (have been/will be) established. The joint working group will receive reports from and monitor and report progress to, the national implementation committee. A project

manager (has been/will be appointed) and will report to the joint working group. *(The specific role and function of the joint working group and the project manager could be indicated (see Chapter 4). In addition, if a Centre for Nurse Education is established, its role in relation to pre-registration nurse education could also be specified.)*

6. **Student Health and Security Screening:**
   All successful applicants who are offered places on the Degree programme will be required to undergo a medical assessment, screening and, if necessary, vaccination prior to the first clinical placement in accordance with the policies of (third-level institution) and (health service provider). The list of potential students' names will also be presented for Garda clearance.

7. **Registration:**
   Each student will be required to register with (third-level institution) for the duration of the Degree programme.

8. **Programme Content:**
   8.1 The programme will meet the requirements of EU Directives 77/453/EEC as amended by Directive 89/595/EEC and will comply with the terms of any relevant legislation or EU Directives and/or Regulations in force from time to time.
   8.2 The location of the theoretical elements of the programme will be principally at X in (third-level institution).

9. **Clinical Placements:**
   9.1 The type and duration of clinical placements for nursing students are as required by An Bord Altranais and arrangements for the clinical placements will be agreed between the Course Leader of (third-level institution) and the (Director of Nursing), (health service provider). *(The agreed arrangements with regard to the allocation function in the third-level institution and the health service provider (see Chapter 6) could be included here.)*

   9.2 The (Director of Nursing), (health service provider), has responsibility for matters relating to clinical placements in so far as they impact on patient care. (Third-level institution) accepts that the (Director of Nursing), (health service provider), will ensure that the clinical placements comply with the agreed placement programme drawn up by the (third-level institution) and comply with the rules of An Bord Altranais and the terms of any relevant legislation or EU Directives and/or Regulations in force from time to time.

   9.3 In planning the programme schedule, arrangements will be made to ensure that the optimum number of nursing students (1st, 2nd and 3rd year) are allocated to the clinical area at any one time so as to allow maximum supervision of students and to optimise the benefit from clinical placements. The first clinical placement will not take place until after X weeks of the first theory (foundation) course component/module are completed.

   9.4 *(This section could include the agreed amounts of reflective time to be allowed to nursing students whilst on supernumerary and rostered clinical placements.)*

10. **Assessment Methodologies and Examinations:**
The regulations governing the conduct and assessment of the Degree examinations will be determined by the (Department/School/Centre/Faculty) Committee as approved by the (third-level institution Academic Council/Board/awarding authority). External examiners will be appointed according to the regulations of (third-level institution Academic Council/Board/awarding authority) and in accordance with the guidelines on standards of An Bord Altranais. (Third-level institution) will be responsible for the conduct of clinical assessments, which will be undertaken in partnership with (health service provider).

11. **Academic Approval/Accreditation:**
The Degree programme has been approved/accredited by (third-level institution Academic Council/Board/awarding authority). Any changes in the programme will be subject to (third-level institution)'s approval/accreditation processes, which are designed to ensure that the programme's academic and professional status meets national and international standards.

12. **Student Welfare and Code of Conduct:**
A Joint Disciplinary Committee has been (will be) established (as soon as possible). It will be chaired by an agreed person. Its first task will be to synchronise the disciplinary regulations and procedures of (third-level institution) and (health service provider).

Students will be expected, while on clinical placement, to comply with relevant standards laid down by the An Bord Altranais Code of Conduct for registered nurses, and the disciplinary code of (health service provider).

Breaches of this Code will be referred, in the first instance, to the Joint Disciplinary Committee composed of selected members from the joint working group (in Section 5 above) representing the views of (third-level institution) and (health service provider).

Information on the role and function of the Joint Disciplinary Committee, and details of the Code of Conduct, will be set out in the handbook to be provided for all students, which will be prepared by the Joint Disciplinary Committee, for approval by the Department/School/Centre/Faculty Committee.

13. **Joint Appointments:**
(This section could refer to the mechanisms in place to facilitate joint appointments and other innovative strategies to enhance partnership between third-level institutions and health service providers as recommended in Chapter 6.)

14. **Review:**
This Memorandum of Understanding will be subject to regular review by both parties acting in consultation. In the absence of either party requesting a review, the text of this Memorandum of Understanding shall remain in effect.

15. **Notice to Terminate the Agreement:**
(Health service provider) and (third-level institution) each undertakes to give not less than X years' formal notice of their intention to withdraw from the arrangements as described in this Memorandum of Understanding.

(health service provider)

_____   _____   _____
Chief Executive Officer   Director of Nursing   Date

(third-level institution)

_____   _____   _____
Secretary/relevant   Director of (Department/   Date
Administrator/Dean of   School/Centre/Faculty of Nursing/
(Health Sciences/Medicine/   Nursing and Midwifery)
Science)

Appendix 4

Domains of Competence[39]

1. Professional and Ethical Practice

2. Assessment, Intervention and the Integration
   of Knowledge

3. Communication Skills

4. Organisation of Work (Management and
   Leadership)

5. Development, Education, Teaching and
   Reflective Practice

[39] These domains are currently being developed by C. Griffin and An Bord Altranais. They will evolve and change over time. The role of competencies in curriculum design for the nursing degree programme is discussed in Chapter 5.

Appendix 5

Calculation of Health and Education Sector Costs, 2002

1. Health Sector Costs, 2002

Salaries of Nurse Tutors and Clinical Placement Co-ordinators

Number of Nurse Tutors in 2002 (Projected by DoHC)	=	225	
Number of Clinical Placement Co-ordinators in 2002 (Projected by DoHC)	=	150	

Nurse Tutor, Max. Salary Scale 1 Oct 2000	=	£33,029	
Clinical Placement Co-ordinator Max. Salary Scale 1 Oct 2000	=	£29,912	

Pay Inflators: 5.5% in 2001 and 4% in 2002

Nurse Tutor, Max. Salary Scale 1 Oct 2002	=	£36,239x225	= **£8.2m**
Clinical Placement Co-ordinator Max. Salary Scale 1 Oct 2002	=	£32,819x150	= **£4.9m**

Third Level Costs and Fees

DoHC Provision 2000	=	£5.2m
Non-Pay Inflators = 3.5% in 2001 and 2.3% in 2002		
DoHC Provision 2002	=	**£5.5m**

Student Maintenance Grant

Grant in 2000	=	£3,325	
Non-Pay Inflators = 3.5% in 2001 and 2.3% in 2002			
Grant in 2002	=	£3,520	
Provided for	x	4,500	Students
		£15.8m	

Book Grant

Grant in 2001	=	£300	
Non-Pay Inflator = 2.3% in 2002			
Grant in 2002	=	£307	
	x	1,500	Students
		£0.5m	

Meals

£3.6m in 1998 for 3,000 students

Spend per student in 1998	=	£1,200	
Non-Pay Inflators = 3% in 1999, 6% in 2000, 3.5% in 2001 and 2.3% in 2002			
Spend per student in 2002	=	£1,387	
	x	4,500	Students
		£6.2m	

Student Salaries

Student Salaries in 1998	=	£2.3m

Pay Inflators 1998 to 2000 = 20%, 5.5% in 2001 and 4% in 2002

Student Salaries in 2002	=	**£3.0m**

Miscellaneous Items[40]   =   £0.6m

Non-Pay Inflators = 3% in 1999, 6% in 2000, 3.5% in 2001 and 2.3% in 2002

Miscellaneous Items in 2002	=	**£0.7m**

2. Education Sector Costs, 2002

Cost of Third Level Academic Programme
Unit Costs (HEA Inflators)

Pay Inflation 1998 to 2000	=	21%
Non-Pay Inflation 1998 to 2000	=	9%

Usual Pay / Non-Pay Breakdown = 75 / 25

Unit Cost Estimate 1998 Prices

Academic Year = £5,000   **Clinical year = £1,500**

Inflation to 2000   Inflation to 2000

£5,000 x 75% x 1.21	=	£4,538	£1,500 x 75% x 1.21	=	£1,361
£5,000 x 25% x 1.09	=	£1,362	£1,500 x 25% x 1.09	=	£ 409

Inflated to 2002   **Inflated to 2002**

(£4,538 + 5.5%) + 4%	=	£4,979	(£1,361 + 5.5%) + 4%	=	£1,493
(£1,362 + 3.5%) + 2.3%	=	£1,442	(£409 + 3.5%) + 2.3%	=	£ 433
Total	=	**£6,421**	**Total**	=	**£1,926**

Average Unit Cost = [(£6,421 x 3 years) + £1,926] / 4 years   =   £5,298[41]

                                                                 x   6,000   Students

Cost of Third-Level Academic Programme in 2002   =   **£31.8m**

---

[40] It was estimated that 50% of miscellaneous items associated with the diploma were offset costs.
[41] In Chapter 7 this figure is rounded to £5,300.

Rostered Clinical Placement

Formula = [n/2 x (80% First Year Salary)] + 22% + 12.5% + 20%

(22% for premium payments, 12.5% for PRSI, 20% for statutory and study leave)

n = 1,500 students

First Year Salary = £16,629 Salary Scale 1 Oct 2000

Pay Inflators: 5.5% in 2001 and 4% in 2002

First year Salary = £18,246 in 2002

750 x (14,597 + £3,211 + £1,825 + £2,919)   =   £16.9m

Student Maintenance Grant

4,500 Students

General Pattern = 40% Eligible, of which 75% at non-adjacent rate and 25% at adjacent rate

2000 / 2001 Grant Rates:

Adjacent = £705

Non-Adjacent = £1,765

Service Fee = £290 (Relieved for both sets of grant holders)

Non-Pay Inflators = 3.5% in 2001 and 2.3% in 2002

2002 / 2003 Grant Rates (rounded):		Numbers of Students	
Adjacent = £745	x	450 =	£335,250
Non-Adjacent = £1,870			
	x	1350 =	£2,524,500
Service Fee = £305 (Relieved for both sets of grant holders)	x	1800 =	£549,000
			£3.4m

References

An Bord Altranais (1994) *The Future of Nurse Education and Training in Ireland*. Dublin: An Bord Altranais.

An Bord Altranais (1999) *Requirements and Standards for Nurse Registration Education Programmes*. Dublin: An Bord Altranais.

An Bord Altranais (2000) *The Scope of Nursing and Midwifery Practice Framework*. Dublin: An Bord Altranais.

Carney, M. (1999) "An Analysis of the Costing of the Registration/Diploma in Nursing in the Republic of Ireland". Unpublished internal Forum briefing paper. Dublin: School of Nursing and Midwifery, University College Dublin.

Council of European Communities (1989) "Council Directive (89/595/EEC)". *Official Journal of the European Communities*, L341, Vol. 32, 23 November 1989.

Creedon, S. and Savage, E. (2000) "An Examination of Clinical Placements in Preparation for the Undergraduate BSc Nurse Education Programme scheduled to commence in 2002". Unpublished internal Forum briefing paper. Cork: Department of Nursing Studies, National University of Ireland, and Cork.

Dunn, S. and Burnett, B. (1995) "The development of a clinical learning environment scale". *Journal of Advanced Nursing*, 22: 1166-1173.

Government of Ireland (1999) *Commission on the Points System: Final Report and Recommendations*. Dublin: Stationery Office.

Government of Ireland (1998) *Report of the Commission on Nursing: A Blueprint for the Future*. Dublin: Stationery Office.

Joyce, P. (2000) *Curriculum Design Principles*. Dublin: Faculty of Nursing, Royal College of Surgeons in Ireland. www.nursingeducationforum.ie

McCarthy, M. (2000) *Creating and Maintaining a Clinical Learning Environment*. Dublin: School of Nursing and Midwifery Studies, Trinity College Dublin. www.nursingeducationforum.ie

McNamara, M. (2000) *The Recruitment and Selection of Nursing Students*. Dublin: Nursing Careers Centre, An Bord Altranais. www.nursingeducationforum.ie

National University of Ireland (1999) *An NUI Qualifications Framework for Lifelong Learning: Access, Progression and Transfer*. Dublin: National University of Ireland.

Quinn, F. (1997) *The Principles and Practice of Nurse Education*. 3rd edition. Cheltenham: Stanley Thornes (Publishers) Ltd.

School of Nursing and Midwifery Studies (2000) "Evaluation and Quality Improvement". Unpublished internal Forum briefing paper. Dublin: Trinity College Dublin.

Simons, H., Clarke, J. B., Gobbi, M., Long, G., Mountford, M. and Wheelhouse, C. (1998) *Nurse Education and Training Evaluation in Ireland. Independent External Evaluation. Final Report*. Southampton: University of Southampton.

World Health Organisation (1999) *Nurses and Midwives for Health, A WHO European Strategy for Nursing and Midwifery Education*. Copenhagen: World Health Organisation.